T0072327

DARWIN'S HEART

Morris Weiss, Jr MD, FACP, FACC

authorHOUSE®

AuthorHouse™
1663 Liberty Drive
Bloomington, IN 47403
www.authorhouse.com
Phone: 833-262-8899

Published by AuthorHouse   04/17/2023

ISBN: 979-8-8230-0499-2 (sc)
ISBN: 979-8-8230-0498-5 (e)

Library of Congress Control Number: 2023906077

Print information available on the last page.

Any people depicted in stock imagery provided by Getty Images are models, and such images are being used for illustrative purposes only. Certain stock imagery © Getty Images.

This book is printed on acid-free paper.

Author's Statement:

My goal is to show that the symbolic heart is an important and vital consideration in the care and treatment of patients with heart disease and that it must be given equal consideration with the heart's function as a pump.

As an example, a woman whose husband died shortly after the implantation of an artificial heart insisted that what remained of his actual heart be replaced in his chest before he was buried. In her mind his actual heart was a part of his whole being. These thoughts were not unique to her but were an accumulation of cultural thoughts and beliefs from the beginning of time.

As the symbolic heart is examined here, we learn the heart has had meaning, symbolically, throughout the ages. Every culture has interpreted it differently but, in every culture, it has been understood as a vital and meaningful part of the whole person.

CONTENTS

A NOTE FROM THE AUTHOR

My father was a cardiologist, but I started my medical education in the 1950s assuming that I would treat children. I had been a camp counselor in my teens, and after my junior year in medical school I was the athletic director at the summer camp I had attended as a child. While interning at the Pennsylvania hospital founded by Benjamin Franklin, I was sent, as were all interns, to the Philadelphia Children's Hospital for a six-week pediatric rotation. The Pennsylvania Hospital interns were given the least complicated and yet hardest jobs on the service: I spent my rotation in an outpatient clinic treating Cooley's anemia and leukemia patients. At that time, most of these children would not live to become teenagers. From my years at camp, I had somehow imagined all kids were eight or nine years old, playing baseball and, at worst, breaking a bone. But that was not how it was in the hospital, of course. The pediatric rotation was very emotionally trying, and I had to look for my passion in a different age group. Fortunately, a Fellowship in Hypertension at the University of Pennsylvania was offered to me, and I discovered my interest in adult heart disease. The doctors on the academic track were competitive and research-based, and a path to academic medicine was open to me, but it meant two years dissecting rat hearts. I wasn't excited by rat hearts—it was the human heart that captivated me. In 1960, I instead began a two-year private service residency in internal medicine at Washington University. When my father had a heart attack on a plane trip in 1962, I was able to join him at the end of my residency in his cardiology practice in June of that year, taking it over when he died six months later.

Throughout my life as a physician and as a student of archaeology, I have made an effort to understand, even if only generally, how various civilizations throughout history have understood "the pump." Many people theorized about the heart's physical context, but until recently, that physical context was continually grounded in an equally weighty symbolic and emotional understanding of this crucial organ. My goal is to explore with you the story of the symbolic heart by teasing out from diverse civilizations, societies, and individuals this archetypical part of our being, one recognized as such long before the heart was identified as a pump with anatomical, mechanical, and histochemical properties. We need science to repair muscle and valves, but truly restorative care cannot be restricted to statistical evaluation alone. While this book will not be long enough to explore all the minutiae and interesting trivia surrounding the heart— rather than long, ponderous footnotes it will, however, provide signposts to further readings—I hope it will provide a working introduction to the symbolic heart's importance and its evolution throughout history. This is one of the many ways that I have been able to understand how best to provide balanced care for my charges.

PREFACE

This book examines how various civilizations have understood the "pump." Understanding this historical environment will allow physicians to know how to provide better care for our patients.

While working in medicine, I have also been lucky enough to be able to pursue my interest in ancient history and archaeology, whenever time and opportunity have allowed. As an archaeologist, I have had the opportunity to excavate at important sites in the Classical world. I have seen the changes made in how excavations are approached, from my readings of nineteenth-century archaeologists, through the first digs I worked on in the mid-1970s, to twenty-first-century approaches. The early archaeologists were great generalists and looked at the big picture, but as time has progressed, excavation techniques have regressed into reductionism. We have made the technical advances necessary to analyze a four-by-four-foot square in the greatest detail, looking deep into the layers of soil and compiling information on each particle. But as rich as this information is, it does not tell us the dig's complete story. The great archaeologist Jacquetta Hawkes in her magnum opus, *The World of the Past*, warns about not forgetting the "big picture." Even in 1963, the price of our race toward specialization was becoming apparent across many fields. What she and the renowned cardiologist Dr. Paul Dudley White each wrote about grappling with both the data in front of us and the big picture that surrounds us has profoundly affected my thinking.

I have spent my career as a practicing cardiologist where artificial hearts have been implanted. These devices, despite their mechanical triumphs, have often failed to live up to emotional expectations.

Grieving patients and their families have primordial responses. In the evolution of *Homo sapiens* the heart is much more than a muscular pump. Ancient societies of which we have some knowledge universally acknowledge the heart as the repository of human emotion. Poets, composers, writers, and even our religious leaders inform us of the power of the heart's love and its healing properties. Charles Darwin claimed the power of reproducing and appreciating music existed in humans long before the power of speech arrived. Ancients understood their hearts, not in any diseased, physical state but out of millennia of cultural experience.

INTRODUCTION

In the desert
I saw a creature, naked, bestial,
Who, squatting upon the ground,
Held his heart in his hands,
And ate of it.
I said, "Is it good, friend?"
"It is bitter—bitter," he answered;

"But I like it,
"Because it is bitter,
"And because it is my heart."
                                    —Stephen Crane, "In the Desert"

It is only with the heart that one can see rightly; what is
essential is invisible to the eye.
                                    —Antoine de Saint-Exupéry

The heart has its reasons, which reason knows nothing of.
                                    —Blaise Pascal

Bacchus opens the gate of the heart.
                                                —Horace

Blue moon,
You saw me standing alone,
Without a dream in my heart,
Without a love of my own.
                                    —Richard Rodgers and Lorenz Hart

Bernardo: 'Tis now struck twelve; get thee to bed, Francisco.
Francisco: For this relief much thanks. 'Tis bitter cold, and I am sick at heart.

—Shakespeare, *Hamlet*

Di klainer hartz nemt arum di groisseh velt.
The heart is small and embraces the whole wide world.

—Yiddish proverb

"Find whatever is left of my husband's heart and put it back inside his chest." In death, a widow's husband has only a hollow space in his chest. The artificial heart that could not save her husband's life has been removed. She wants his original heart back in its place.

I am a cardiologist, and this story has had a profound effect on me.

The year 1628 saw the publication of William Harvey's *De Motu Cordis* (On the motion of the heart). This small volume is arguably the most important treatise in the history of medicine, providing for Western Europe the first outline of the workings of the cardiovascular system as a whole. Since that momentous year, both society and science have been fascinated with the chemistry, biophysics, mechanics, and genetics of the heart and blood vessels. As a result of this scientific preoccupation, we've forgotten the symbolic significance of the heart. The organic and symbolic hearts, both crucial to us in their separate ways, are entangled like a Celtic knot of flowers, leaves, stems, and mystical creatures. The dualistic nature of the heart may seem extraneous to cardiology, but I began to feel the need to understand the often-overlooked symbolic role of the heart even before that widow so insightfully and instinctually might have called upon his twenty-first-century doctors for her husband's absent heart.

The heart as a reflection of history, and loss, and the ways cardiologists can too easily overlook the symbolic hearts that secretly drive us have always concerned me. Come with me, for a moment, back to a night early in my career as a cardiologist. I'm sitting at 2:00 a.m. in the most intensive of intensive care units—the beds with open-heart surgery patients, not just those undergoing coronary bypass, but those waiting on transplants. Watching over these patients in the middle of that 1970s night, I am reminded of the youthful Edward Gibbon as he sat one eighteenth-century evening in the ruins of the Roman Forum. He envisioned the most glorious sight of the triumphant parades honoring Roman generals and emperors. On that evening the Forum around Gibbon was a melancholy scene of fallen marble blocks, with vines and brambles covering 1,500 years of detritus, become only a feeding ground of swineherds' animals. Edward Gibbon saw the whole of the place's past in these unpretentious broken fragments.

Back in the 1970s ICU, the limp stethoscope hanging on my shoulders is a sign of how I feel, but I am alert to the carnage surrounding me. My patient is the epicenter. A ceiling light illuminates the bed with innumerable wires, tubes, mechanical devices, and monitoring equipment attached to and penetrating the body. Surrounding the bed and spilling out into the nurses' station are sheets and used packaging containers, discarded ampules and syringes. The scene reminds me of what carnage must've appeared in Rome after the Goths' pillage, or at the sack of Troy by the Greeks. The patient is a good candidate for surgery, and will have his life extended if the high-tech operation is successful—but at what emotional and physical cost? I provide this care to this patient because life is our most precious commodity, and I have a medical and religious obligation to preserve life. The preservation of life takes precedence over all other obligations in our world of medicine, but perhaps, in looking only at the picture before us, we miss the rich parades of our patients' histories and the tools they might need to grieve, or flourish, or heal. I first conceived of this book while viewing this ICU event. The subject has exercised me for years.

Imagine a man at the end of his life is dying of congestive heart failure. The heart has failed as a pump, the organ's primary function. Its chambers are dilated and no longer thrust an adequate volume of blood through his arteries and veins, and thus can no longer sustain the lungs, kidneys, heart, and life itself. He's lingered for months, receiving the best medical treatment scientific medicine can offer, but he is now essentially bedridden. After much discussion with the patient and his wife, they consent to implantation of an artificial heart. The operation is a success, but his post-operative course is protracted. It starts with transient heart failure and finally ends with a paralytic stroke, leaving the patient in a virtual vegetative state. His mechanical heart pumps, but his life is over. The artificial heart is disconnected.

In the wake of the surgery, the patient and his wife express regret that they consented to the operation. The artificial heart is removed at autopsy, as usual at a recipient's death, for study. But in this case, to the surprise of the medical experts working with this couple, the patient's wife insists the cardiac surgeon find what is left of the original organ—presumably preserved in a formaldehyde bottle in the pathology laboratory—and replace it inside the patient before he was buried.

For a bereaved spouse, their final consolation might be that their partner would be with their "human heart." It is these possible reactions that have a profound effect on me. Halfway through my career I realized, even though I am a scientific cardiologist in the twenty-first century, I needed to study in greater detail and depth the emotional heart.

We, as scientists and as healers, have missed the mark. Every patient who is considered a candidate for an implantable heart must be provided with the informed-consent information from the artificial heart's manufacturer. This information addresses the scientific aspects of the surgery as it should. It cannot address the spiritual, religious, emotional, and family considerations. This important aspect of patient care is not today given sufficient consideration. I think there is a need for pastoral care. Consent, to be "informed," must include both the scientific as well as the holistic mental and social considerations.

My medical life has been greatly influenced by a small book published in 1967 by the great American cardiologist Paul Dudley White, entitled *Hearts: Their Long Follow-Up.* The coauthor, Helen Donovan, was Dr. White's long-time secretary. Dr. White was a brilliant and often publicly active physician, treating President Eisenhower's 1955 heart attack and, in a press briefing, informing and reassuring the country more effectively than the president's appointed physician. He also ran a clinic out of Massachusetts General Hospital that treated people from all walks of life throughout his career. With Ms. Donovan's assistance, Dr. White describes the cardiology cases in patients he had followed from twenty to fifty years. He recounts how these patients, by all rights, should have died years before, but they survived, and many led essentially normal lives. His work implies that long-term follow-up care in individual cases is more important and often more revealing than the more publicized short-term, controlled scientific studies of large groups that only follow a patient for three months to two years.

All physicians have long-term patients who, by all measured parameters, should have passed away or been severely impaired, but nevertheless survive and enjoy a full life. My experience is that these enduring survivors have an internal equanimity that promotes healing, and this equanimity seems in a vague, ill-defined way to be controlled by cultural features I can only imagine. Dr. White's brief monograph and the clinical circumstances of that early night in the cardiac ICU, as well as a widow's impassioned plea, piqued my curiosity, pushing me to try to better understand the cultural significance of the heart.

Even before that night in the ICU when I wondered how our patients would approach their new lives after emerging from the wreckage of their lifesaving surgeries, I had been a student of history where and when I could be. My avocation is archaeology. I have learned a little about the details of reconstructing past lives out of the potshards buried under centuries of dirt, and there is much we can learn from the historical record of those who came before us. To understand how we have been shaped, however unwittingly, by our relationship to the symbolic heart, I have tried to tease out of the archaeological records and what remains of the earliest images the thoughts about the heart as developed by our distant ancestors. The heart is recognized and dreamed of by the earliest of our ancestors. While we often speak of how our understanding of the heart as mechanical pump came to be, that understanding is, we will see, inevitably tied up in our emotional response to all the heart represents, at all stages of history—even our own.

Whether in cardiology or in archaeology, my concern is that we are becoming much too specialized and reducing smaller and smaller our focus in specialization. In a hundred years, they will laugh at our fixation with the .10 mm size of the lumen—the inside diameter—of a small coronary artery, as described by the modern-day magic of intracoronary sonography, but now this is all we can accomplish. Scientific reductionism is fraught with hazard, since we look at only a minute area instead of the larger picture. We are victims of the philosopher Husserl's phenomenological limitations, instead of beneficiaries of the generalist Paul Dudley White, who fought against this tide in medicine. Dr. White wanted to keep the field of vision wide and not narrow. The heart has many cultural ramifications, and whether or not we acknowledge them, they influence how patients view their disease. Patients do not look at the cardiac cellular metabolism to understand its function, but intuitively understand their heart from millennia of spoken and unspoken cultural circumstance. We need science, of course, but we cannot be chained to every chi-square conclusion that the strictly calculated statistical model outlines for us.

There must be more to the evolution of the *Homo sapiens* heart. The efficiency of the physical, mechanical pump that moves our blood is not the only measure of our long relationship with this central organ of our bodies. We speak effusively of the art of medicine, but the integration of science and intuition is still needed as I pass from bed to bed in the hospital, and as I move, every twenty minutes or so, from examining room to examining room in my office. Patient care involves not just my knowledge of ventricles and vessels, but also my awareness of my patients' fears and goals for their health and for their lives. We relate to our hearts not just through cholesterol level and electrical signals—our hearts are also full of aches, and love, and the beats we hear when we hold our loved ones close. The symbolic heart has long been recognized as a repository of good and evil. The nature of human evil is so pervasive that we have developed the ability to destroy our species, in multiple ways and by multiple paths. I do not recognize any other species with such distemper. My hope is that coming to an understanding and appreciation of the archetypical heart can be of benefit even beyond the personal, individual level, and that this understanding can grow to be a counterattack to the evil lurking so often in some hidden cranny of our collective brain.

René Descartes, in the early seventeenth century, enunciated dualism, separating body from mind. His mechanistic theory of organ function produced, over the centuries, the concept of reductionism. This approach fosters the illusion that an understanding of details alone can provide the most accurate answers to our questions. Much of contemporary medical research is working at the level of molecules and genes. I do not reject the notion of reductionism—after all, I'm a practicing cardiologist who specializes by necessity in the function of the heart—but this essay will view the heart from a holistic and prescientific vista, in order to return crucial elements of the bigger picture to our awareness.

The historical record of the symbolic heart is remarkably long and wide-ranging. Prehistoric cave painters in France and Spain depicted the life they understood in the art they created. From there, the record is thin, until the cuneiform writing of the early Mesopotamian civilizations provides another window for us. Then the Egyptians give us a sudden burst of detail, as their hieroglyphic writings reveal much of how they conceived of the heart, medically and spiritually. These civilizations influenced the ideas of the ancient Greeks and Romans, whose works in turn influenced Judeo-Christian thought. Meanwhile, across the globe in Mesoamerica and in East Asia, the heart was also being contemplated, studied, and folded into yet more ancient worldviews. Much of the physical and spiritual conception of the heart was gained, then lost, and hidden from view over more recent millennia, until 1628's crucial, foundational analysis by William Harvey of the physical processes by which the circulatory system and the heart work in unison.

I must mention some caveats here at the outset of this journey. My observations may lack profundity—but that is for the reader to decide. As a historian, I am an amateur who has read widely and in a cheerful spirit. I have not read the original manuscripts in the many languages encountered. To compensate for this I have used only the most recognized specialist in each culture writing in English, or the most reliable English translation of the ancient works. Just as my patients may need to understand the working of their hearts at the broadest levels as they start on their journeys to recovery and health, I have confined myself here to understanding the broadest picture of the history of the symbolic heart. I have navigated this voluminous historical material in shallow waters, as not to drown.

Darwin posits that music and art arise for humans before speech does. Much as art provides those first, primal connections between us, art also provides the earliest window into the most ancient of our symbolic hearts.

THE SYMBOLIC HEART

Symbols underscore much of our experiences throughout our lives, despite our modern reliance on the rational understanding of mechanical functions, especially when we consider the health and function of our hearts. We know what *heart-shaped* means—two lobes, and flat—and when we say a thing is heart-shaped, we do not mean it looks like the four-chambered fist-shaped organ beating inside our chests, unless of course we are standing in my office. To the cardiologist, *heart-shaped* may evoke a different image than the cartoon we think of on Valentine's Day, but even the cardiologist must remember the symbolic weight attached to that cartoon.

A symbol—for example, any of the many meanings that the cartoon heart drawing may imply—is complementary to the rational world of concepts. The heart as an organ is a sign, not a symbol. Andreas Vesalius and William Harvey, when they described the function of the heart and captured it for the world to study, turned the heart from a symbol to a sign. But, as I learned from the story of the widow who wanted her husband's heart placed back again in his body at his death, even four hundred years after Harvey's revelations, the symbolic function of the heart has not gone away—it remains eternal.

The symbolic heart has many images, neither rational nor irrational. Heart symbols, like all symbols, point to the unknown. Once the meaning of a symbol is known it becomes a sign. As a physician I always respond to signs, as symptoms and test results and other metrics. This essay, however, is about the persistence of the hidden symbolic value of the heart.

Like the writer who creates symbols with which to define our fears of mortality or our yearning to love, and then transforms them through language into signs, and like the actor who then returns the symbolic weight to the words as they are spoken aloud and imbued with feelings, or the reader who is moved by those words to glimpse the symbols they address, I hope in this essay to highlight the symbolic meanings the heart has carried through our collective past, to make of that meaning a sign that can allow those of us who work in the sign-filled world of medicine a route back to the best treatment of our patients—to be able to address their concerns about not just their mechanical hearts, but also their symbolic fears and hopes.

Study of the symbolic heart leads the scholar hither and yon. The heart's mechanical purpose was not comprehensively defined until William Harvey's 1628 monograph, but humans have been aware of the heart as a vital force, and vital organ, since our earliest artistic records, if not from time immemorial.

What is the story of the evolution of the heart as a symbol? The conventional two-lobed heart symbol is recognized around the world. This ideogram is used to express the idea of the heart in its metaphorical symbolic sense as the center of emotion, including affection and love, especially but not exclusively romantic love.

The earliest depiction of our modern two-lobed heart shape is found in a Paleolithic cave in France. In 2008, I chose to visit six caves in the Dordogne region of France where the first cave art was discovered. Even these mysterious humans, our ancestors who first left records of their art and thus their thoughts and cares, though not entirely decipherable, reveal to us that on some level they too assigned some crucial respect to the heart in its two-lobed potential.

Abbé Breuil in his classic tome from 1952, *Quatre cents siècles d'art pariétal* (*Four Hundred Years of Cave Art*), reproduces a drawing of an ancient elephant with an almost modern valentine-shaped heart drawn on the left front flank in the chest area. This drawing in the Pindar Cave, located in the valley of Pimiango, Spain, on a plateau near the sea, has been dated to the Magdalenian period, and was drawn, we think, sometime between 11,000 to 7000 BCE.

The placement of the heart in this drawing is both symbolic and anatomically precise. While contemplating the ancient impulses that may lie behind this drawing, I became curious. Was the placement's apparent accuracy merely my own uninformed or biased assumption? I obtained from a veterinary library an anatomic atlas of this species. A reader peels back each page to see the anatomical structure, beginning with the skin through layers into the internal organs. One can see from this anatomical illustration that in that ancient animal painting, if a spear were to be thrust through the symbol, if driven in deep enough, the tip of this spear would penetrate the depicted animal's heart and aorta.

This heart shape predates by at least ten thousand years the reappearance of this form in our historical period.

The modern student's attempt to focus on the symbolic heart first requires a definition of terms so often loosely tossed about in the vast accumulation of literature about the symbolic heart. Our first task is to define *archetype*, because the major writers on the symbolic heart have almost all universally used the phrase *archetypical heart* to discuss the heart in its symbolic, rather than mechanical, form.

The Greek word *archetype* is best translated as "beginning pattern"; the phrase "first form" is also used but is cumbersome. Perhaps a better definition is "prototype." The prototype or beginning pattern is a primordial image or character, best understood in this case as an entity occurring throughout literature that remains consistent enough to be considered a universal concept. I must confess in the beginning of this discussion of archetypes that I'm a linear thinker and wrapping my arms around this very nonlinear subject is difficult, but because understanding the history of the symbolic heart is key to any understanding of our modern heart, I will give it a try.

Archaeologists have uncovered many artifacts revealing that the earliest humans were quite advanced in their emotional makeup. Even for those early humans, complex symbolism was deeply embedded in their psyche. Artistry, as action that involves work that is outside of the immediate needs of food and shelter, arises early in our prehistoric story. A forty-thousand-year-old flute made from a vulture bone has been found in a German cave, and animal cave paintings in France date from twelve thousand to thirty-four thousand years ago. What came before this bone flute and these cave paintings? Though we do not have many tangible artifacts, we have many theories. To understand the possible beginnings of the role of our archetypical heart, I've chosen to focus on the theories of Carl G. Jung, the Swiss psychologist who studied under Sigmund Freud, and Jung's student James Hillman, who also studied under Henry Corbin, a scholar of both western and eastern philosophical thought.

Jung formulated the theory of collective unconsciousness, describing this as, in many ways, a driving force for all of human culture. Jung proposed that this collective unconscious houses the archetypes that we use, across all cultures and throughout history, as implicit maps of who we can conceive of being. In the unconscious are found the basic fairy tales, as exemplified by the Grimm Brothers' collections, and Greek epic poetry, including the *Iliad* and the *Odyssey*. In these stories, we find hero and antihero of Jung's collective unconscious, and they are also found embedded in our psyche, as often expressed in writing, art, and even in our dreams.

Jung felt religion and religious symbols had an archetypical origin and explanation. His archetypes are always instinctive, and with universal characters they express our behavior in the images society creates. This collective corpus is present in prelogical thought, but when expressed in literature and plastic arts, the artist views these sensations and feelings and expresses them so that less artistic persons, like myself, can enjoy the symbols that the artist has rendered back to the audience through the externalization of the art itself.

Parallels between science and myth do exist and are recognized both inside and outside of Jung's sphere of thought. The ancient Greeks, whom we must always refer back to, had elaborate myths related to physics and medicine, to name but two sciences, that are paradigms of the human world. Over the past two and a half millennia, these myths have been replaced by new knowledge, but they were the originators of science as we now know and practice it. The Greeks loved their stories and venerated their work, but they also knew gods were myths themselves derived from long-dead kings and heroes.

Ultimately, Jungian psychology says these unconscious patterns, images, and ideas are inherited from our ancestors, beginning at least 250,000 years ago, when modern *Homo sapiens* entered the greater world from Africa. If indeed Jung is correct and these unconscious patterns are embedded in our genes, their origin undoubtedly predates any conceptions of modern man. This genetic concept resonates with me because of my medical background. The genetic mechanism of conscious and unconscious thought form the totality of our mind. They are two halves of the whole. The unconscious part of our thoughts consists of symbols or instinctual patterns and the conscious thoughts are signs or logical patterns. In this modern world, devoted to rational thought and rationalism itself, we can only with difficulty and often anxiety imagine anything not explained by logic, which we call common sense.

From 1914 to 1930, Jung recorded, revised, and wrote, recopied, and painstakingly illustrated the beginning of his most sophisticated work, *The Red Book*, devoted to the impact of the collective unconscious on himself and on rational thought. In many ways, this work was a repudiation of his mentor Freud's saddling to each individual's unconscious urges all the worst motivations of people's inner lives.

Jung began the book not long after he fell out with Sigmund Freud. Jung agreed with Freud's basic theory that the unconscious mind exists beyond the reach of consciousness and yet influences human behavior. He also believed, however, that Freud's conception of the unconscious as a dark vault of repressed urges and denied emotions was incomplete and unnecessarily negative. Freud focused too much on neurosis. The 1912 publication of Jung's *Psychology of the Unconscious*, which had grown out of his psychoanalysis of heroes and heroines of mythology, folklore, and religion, made the two doctors' different opinions become public. Jung states that in the psychoanalysis of heroes and heroines found in the mythology of Greece, Rome, and other ancient cultures, one could find archetypical concepts that were universal. As he worked on this conception of the unconscious as a collective repository, Jung was simultaneously afraid of torment with hallucinations similar to those suffered by schizophrenic patients. As a result, he produced this book of the unconscious mind. He wrote his *Red Book* in Latin and medieval script and filled it with complex paintings and drawings that involved trees and snakes and demons, designing images similar to the Tibetan paintings that are called mandala.

Some other works that border on this, and that directly or indirectly shaped Jung's thinking here, include Friedrich Wilhelm Nietzsche's *Thus Spoke Zarathustra*, a major influence on Jung. The book describes the rebirth of God in the soul, drawing from many and varied sources including the Bible, the Apocrypha, Gnostic texts, Greek myths, ancient

Egyptian writings, Richard Wagner's *Ring* cycle, Dante Alighieri's *Divine Comedy*. These writers all probed the depths of unconsciousness in myth.

In the book, Jung embarks on a series of adventures and meets with, among others, Elijah, Salome, the serpent, and the devil. He meets people in a castle in the forest, and Jung remarks in the book, "I am really truly in hell," but feels resurrected as time passes. In forging a work not just of psychological analysis but of a primary art itself, Jung—perhaps inadvertently—concretely illustrates his most crucial insight for those attempting to understand the lasting significance of human focus and reverence: the functions in our collective and individual thoughts of symbols and signs. To understand the way the symbolic heart affects our visualization of the mechanical heart, we must fix these ideas, however bewildering, in our minds.

The importance of noting the difference in a sign and a symbol cannot be overemphasized.

As Jung outlines for us, a sign is less than the concept it represents. A symbol inevitably stands for something more than what is merely obvious. If a writer or artist depicts a symbol, it immediately becomes a sign, linked to the artist's conscious thought process. The symbol is always more than the sign. Symbols can be collective or personal, or even both. On the most personal level, a symbol can, of course, be linked only to an individual who is experiencing it in a dream. However, there are, more importantly for this essay, universal symbols. We are frequently taught most universal symbols are of religious origin. The heart—whether in its two-lobed, flat metaphysical shape or in its use in poem, prayer, or song—is also a universal symbol. It is a universal collective symbol and not a wholly modern intentional invention or sign.

As a practicing physician, dealing with the individual patient—the sign of the mechanical heart is the only reality for me and my patient. So while I must avoid abstract ideas that cause me to meander from my mission, I must try to understand the heart as both a sign and a symbol, in order to clarify the sign and still see the ways the symbol can possibly affect each patient. The heart is an organ, like the brain, with other functions of evolutionary development lost in the mists of archaic man. Through studying the symbol's evolution, often in light of our evolving knowledge of the mechanical heart, I will become more harmonious with my patients' anxieties and desires.

For me, the symbolic heart, like all symbols, is nature itself and is neutral. So as we uncover the heart, I expect to find good and evil, light and dark.

I have touched on Carl Jung and established him as originator and developer of the archetypal concept. Jung had many followers and disciples, which can easily confuse the student who is striving to grasp the incredibly complex and dense ideas that he grappled with.

In my attempt to connect the heart to the archetypal scheme, I have chosen to study James Hillman, an American, born in 1926, in Atlantic City, New Jersey, of Jewish and European ancestry. He served in the United States Navy during World War II (1944–46). Eventually, he studied at the Sorbonne in Paris and Trinity College in Dublin, Ireland. In 1959, he earned his PhD at the University of Zurich at the C. G. Jung Institute as an analyst.

Hillman can be broadly described as an archetypal psychologist, in contrast with Jung, an archetypal analyst. Hillman moved from the medical clinic into the world of art, poetry, and mythology—especially of Western civilization. For Hillman and Jung, archetypal forms are all universal. Jung was concerned about the biochemical and genetic basis, as well as the social and personal, of the archetypal form. For Hillman, the ideal forms are more imaginative and poetic in structure. It is through Hillman's emphasis we can begin to understand the cultural heart. For Hillman, all pathology is related to mythology, or our archetypal stories. It makes no difference if the myths are of the Middle Ages, or found in the Brothers Grimm—or in anthologies or ancient Greek epics like the *Iliad* and the *Odyssey*. For Hillman, all of these stories understand the universal nature of archetypal ideas and forms lost in the fog of prehistory as revealed in our memories, dreams, and subconscious reflections.

Hillman says we can be in the world through the heart rather than the head—a reality he saw reflected in the patients he studied. He describes a case in the Psychiatric Institute in Zurich of an elderly lady who said she was dead, for she had lost her heart. Her physician said, "Put your hand on your chest and feel your heart beating. If you can feel it, it must be there." Her answer: "That is not my real heart." The story is used to emphasize Hillman's concept that we can be in the world through our symbolic, poetic heart and not just our head. This woman did not feel connected to the world through her mechanical, beating heart, thus revealing that her feeling of separation from her imagined, symbolic heart was more important in her experience of her own life. This case is the very nature of the concerns I present and the reason for this book. Hillman in his discussion of evil refers to the anesthetized heart that fails to react to life events. This turns the world into gray, amorphous, and monotonous existence, which he described as "the modern condition."

If we can arrive at an understanding of Hillman, we can grasp the heart as a symbol and image. Hillman was a prolific writer. His biography contains at least eighteen full-length books and hundreds of articles and speeches translated into twenty-one languages. For our purposes, his essay "The Thought of the Heart and the Soul of the World," derived from a series of lectures given at the Eranos Conference in Ascona, Switzerland, in 1979, is the most pertinent of his works.

Hillman describes the heart as comprised of three major images as expressed in our culture:

- The Heart of the Lion or Coeur de Lion. This aspect of the heart is a person's strength and passion. Loyalty, compassion, and humanity emanate from this version of the heart.
- The Heart of William Harvey, discoverer of the circulation. This aspect reveals the anatomic heart, simply a gross anatomy organ, with mechanical, biochemical, and electrical properties.
- The Heart of St. Augustine, a Catholic theologian. This aspect treats the heart as the seat of the soul. Here, in this version of the heart, love, sin, and shame reside.

The Heart of the Lion comes to us through folklore and symbols, most particularly the symbol of the sun. The sun makes us think of gold, heat, redness, and kings. The heat, of course, warms us, and from the loving vitality and imaginative thinking emerges. We, as modern thinkers, may see ties between this image and the physical aspects of mustering courage in the face of fear—a blush when speaking out, or the racing pulse of standing firm in the face of a physical threat—but the source of this aspect, for Hillman, resides entirely in the accumulated symbols of our collected religious, mythological, and narrative histories.

The Heart of Harvey is the first experimental verification of the uninterrupted circulation. Ancient Chinese and Egyptian documents discussed the circulation, but no one until William Harvey got it precisely right. Harvey dedicates his 1628 *De Motu Cordis* to King Charles I, and draws an analogy between the roles of the heart and the king, noting how a kingdom must function in an organized and functional manner, as must the heart. For Harvey, the heart is a visual phenomenon and can be held in your hand. This is in contrast to the Heart of the Lion and the Heart of St. Augustine, both of which cannot be seen, held, or measured.

For St. Augustine, the heart is the origin of feeling, the vessel that holds the true interior and secret places of an individual. Despite the religious framework of this aspect, his approach reveals a true philosophical and psychological phenomenon. St. Augustine's insights are the most profound of any theologian and involve the universal concepts of the heart—not just as a treasury of the feelings of Jews, Christians, or Muslims, but as a universal site, where love and misery reside in their imaginal state for all—not in a form modified by religious dogma.

Hillman credits, alongside himself and his mentor Jung, another twentieth-century philosopher, Henry Corbin, as the third member of this herculean triad. Corbin was a philosopher who incorporated Greek philosophy, mainly Platonism, with Islamic mysticism and philosophy. He defines the core of his psychology of spiritualism in his major work *Avicenna and the Visionary Recital*, which established Corbin as a leading European professor of Islamic studies, philosophy, and theology. His expansive work was an important source for Hillman's psychology of archetypes, which further developed the psychology of Carl Jung.

In preparation of this chapter I've read voluminously from textbooks, journals, newspaper articles, and biographies devoted to those who have worked to bring to life the symbolic and spiritual heart.

One evening, I realized that every piece of this vast corpus of works was derivative.

Yes, Freud, Jung, Hillman, and Corbin are the four luminaries of the nineteenth and twentieth centuries, and their work has had far-reaching import. But, when they outlined the history of the heart, they were paraphrasing Greek mythology with an occasional nod to the Brothers Grimm.

They have shown me that, despite their efforts, this overview must return, again, to the histories and artifacts that are the sources of the archetypes Jung and Hillman took such pains to analyze, track, and turn into signs that could be understood not just intuitively but rationally. But, as I have learned from their own emphasis on the distinctive functions of signs and symbols, the symbol always points to the unknowable, indescribable feelings and impulses it is attempting to elucidate. To determine the import of the archetypes we have inherited, we must look again at history to find in our ancient records the thread of our artistic and medical interactions with our always symbolic and often biologic hearts.

So, for me, back to studying the ancient Greeks. I will move on from these psychoanalytical writings (especially those of Hillman, whose sentence structure is cumbersome, and whose strained syntax I will be happy to leave behind).

Because of the lasting nature of their works, the Greeks and Romans have, through the compelling narratives they wove and the records they were able to keep, become our most accessible bridge to the ancient past. Homer's poems the *Iliad* and the *Odyssey*, composed probably in the seventh century BCE about events occurring in around the twelfth century BCE, along with the works of Plato, Aristotle, and other Greek philosophers in the golden era of Athens in the fifth to the fourth century BCE, added their own twists to this ancient knowledge but their work rests on the foundation stones quarried and chiseled into the works of art all Western thought reclines upon.

The Greeks and Romans, despite their long-standing traffic in symbols that they have passed down to us, are not the sole source of our modern two-lobed heart ideogram, though they are one of the realms this symbol passed through on its route to its current shape. Starting from a motif based in the flora that surrounded the artists, the symbol acquired new meanings and refinements as it progressed through the ages.

In the Museum of Kabul in Afghanistan, from pre-Greek, pre-Roman, pre-Christian times, there is a bulbous, baked-clay goblet which dates from the first half of the third millennium BCE. The goblet is decorated with stylized fig leaves with broad stems. This decoration can be found on later ceramics of neighboring cultures. Along with other vegetal decorations, there appear these same fig leaves—and later ivy leaves—which anticipate the modern heart shape.

Approximately one thousand years later these botanic patterns appeared on Cretan clay vessels; fresco painters decorated scenes of figures in Minoan palaces with naturalistically painted tendrils of ivy, leaves that we now think of as heart-shaped.

The Achaeans, heirs of the Minoan culture and bearers of the Mycenaean culture group, adopted the stylized ivy leaf in their ornamentations, and in the later eighth century BCE, Corinthian vase painters depicted these ornaments on the decorative borders of vase paintings and on the handles of vessels. In many cases even grape leaves in this era are portrayed with this same two-lobed, modern heart shape.

This decoration is a foretaste of the metamorphosis of this shape into the later heart symbolism, as it is described in Christian teachings, portraying Jesus as a vine with a divine, unselfish heart.

Continuing in the pre-Christian era in the Mediterranean region, heart-shaped ivy and vine tendrils can be found on vase paintings of Dionysos, the god of wine, frequently in erotic scenes. On Grecian stelae, and later on Roman gravestones, the ivy leaf symbolizes eternal love. This imagery carried over into use on early Christian graves in the catacombs of Rome, which also bear the ivy leaves and vines that represent eternal love, now starting to represent as well the eternal love of early Church teachings.

The final transformation of the ivy leaf into the red playing-card heart of spiritual and physical love took place in parallel with the secularization of the religious heart metaphor into the worldly, courtly heart imagery found in the literature of the Middle Ages. The monasteries that preserved the records and religious works of the Church were the distillery through which the two-lobed ivy leaf took on the features of the heart symbol that we are so familiar with today.

The monastic illustrators, inspired by art and ornamentation of the latter years of antiquity and Roman times, painted trees of life with heart-shaped leaves, perhaps evoking love not only on the spiritual level, but also on the physical, in light of the foundational narrative juxtaposition of the tree of life and the tree of knowledge; in paintings of the twelfth and thirteenth centuries, ivy leaves appeared in love scenes, and before long they were colored in red—the color of warm blood, which had signified good luck, health, and love since prehistoric times.

From then on, the red heart spread quickly across Europe, especially where the Catholic Church held sway. Several facts are responsible for this. While the profanation of the heart-shaped leaf to a symbol of physical love was not approved by the Church, the no-longer-entirely-a-leaf shape also became a symbol of compassion and devotion in both secular and religious art. The adoption of the heart image in the Sacred Heart cult of the Catholic Church was another step in the elevation of the two-lobed heart shape as a symbol of the heart itself, and all that referencing a heart could convey. And finally, the inclusion of the heart in the deck of cards should not be understated: at the end of the fifteenth century, playing cards began to be standardized, especially their symbols. The red heart replaced the goblets found on Italian tarot cards, delineating these cards from tarot's roots, often a more secular tool of divination.

The heart shape was not confined to portrayals of love or gamesmanship alone. At the close of the Middle Ages until the Baroque period, heart-shaped leaves and hearts can be found on Gothic gravestones, calling forth both spiritual love and the eternal life and love that the Romans and early Christians had portrayed with those early ivy-leaf carvings. Later, in the Renaissance and especially in the Baroque Age, the heart on a coat of arms officially stood for eternal faithfulness and courage. Increasingly, painters and sculptors portrayed the human heart in the form of the playing-card heart more often, especially when they wanted to depict erotic or religious subjects.

Because the heart itself had accrued so much symbolic meaning, European spiritual and secular sovereigns often chose a separate grave for their heart in a place that they were fond of during their lives. The urn was often heart-shaped, or the grave was marked by the heart symbol.

The first medical illustrations of the heart, dating from the Middle Ages, were shaped like pinecones or pyramids, and were probably influenced by the description of the organ by the Hippocratic School, by Galen, and later by Arabian doctors, despite various cultural and legal restrictions on human dissection. Later, from the thirteenth to the sixteenth centuries, the organ is depicted in the form derived from the ivy leaf.

The knowledge of anatomy which Hellenic physicians had gained through autopsies had sunk into oblivion during the Middle Ages, which were characterized by strict religious codes and almost universal prohibitions on any postmortem dissections. The anatomists were inspired by artists and book illustrators, and portrayed the heart as an inverted leaf, with the tip bent to the left and the stem symbolizing the arterial tree.

Even the universal genius Leonardo da Vinci used this analogy between the leaf symbol and the realistic shape in his early anatomic sketches.

But even as it reflected limited anatomical knowledge in the western world, the heart symbol retained and even strengthened its symbolic ties to love and faithfulness, both romantic and spiritual. The ring with the heart-shaped ivy leaf held by the divine hand is an ornament symbolizing eternal love, a so-called *corona vitae*—crown of life. This symbol of love beyond death was taken from the ancient Roman world and became Christian symbolism. In sacral art from medieval times on, angels and saints hold their hearts in their hands like playing cards and give them to God as a sign of their self-sacrificing and everlasting love.

Interestingly, the playing-card heart shape also developed under Buddhism—independently of its western metamorphosis—from the leaves of the Bodhi tree, the fig tree under which the Buddha sat through years of meditation to attain enlightenment. But in this case, it transformed into the symbol not of love, but of enlightenment.

Today, across the world, the symbol with the two curves running down to a tip is a pictogram for a whole range of feelings, and has become the emblem of cardiology.

Despite the symbol's ultimate evolution, the prehistoric potters in Afghanistan and the Greek vase painters did not associate the ivy leaf decoration with the heart of ancient times. The vegetal symbol, however, absorbed so much meaning in the course of European cultural history and to the present, it turned into a general, yet exclusive, optically unique symbol of this central organ and, in human consciousness, a hint of the ancient idea of the seat of the soul, of love, and indeed of consciousness and thought.

I should also address the profound influence of Charles Darwin to bolster my idea of the evolutionary influence of the heart on human emotional responses. Darwin is most famous for his prolific writings about biology. In addition to his theory of evolution, he also studied coral reefs, earthworms, and carnivorous plants, always attempting to understand the intricate systems upon which life depends.

Toward the end of his life, Darwin conducted studies on how people recognize the emotion in facial expressions of *Homo sapiens* in more and less technologically advanced societies and in lower animals. This culminated in his 1872 work, *The Expression of the Emotions in Man and Animals*. Darwin reviewed the world literature on the subject and communicated with scientists and nonscientists living in many types of societies in the nineteenth-century British Empire.

The world is indebted to Peter Snyder and neuroscientists at Brown University who discovered, while doing historical research at the University of Cambridge in England, the notes from Darwin's experiment on emotion in a facial expression. Snyder has carefully studied this single blind study conducted at Darwin's home in Kent County, England. Snyder, along with coauthors Rebecca Kaufman, John Harrison, and Paul Maruff, analyzed data (in Darwin's and his wife Emma's handwriting), presenting their analysis in the *Journal of the History of Neurosciences*.

The details of this forgotten experiment are not included in Darwin's 1872 book. A single blind experiment plus Darwin's thoughts, so thoroughly outlined in his book, became the forerunner for an entire field of contemporary neuropharmacology. Sigmund Freud knew of Darwin's theories of the evolutionary origin of emotion and this in turn influenced Jung, Hillman, and Corbin. While Darwin's focus was on facial expressions, his notes encompass, as they must, the entire physical system that produces the changes his experiment is tracking. Without perhaps even knowing it, the great theorist himself alludes to the centrality of the heart as both a symbol of our feelings and a physical instrument that powers our bodies—and so I end this brief diversion on the evolutionary universality of emotion with Darwin's casual comment, from his notes: "Anger causes an increase in the heart rate."

I conclude this chapter with an observation about the interconnected realities of our mechanical and symbolic hearts.

In medieval through to contemporary iconography, the "wounded heart" indicates lovesickness, often showing the heart pierced by an arrow. As a cardiologist I have treated several women—though this can occur as well in men—for the "ultimate broken heart," Takotsubo Syndrome. This syndrome describes a patient with severe chest pain during severe emotional distress with electrocardiograph changes of an acute myocardial infarction, or, in common parlance, a heart attack, but the arteries are open and not blocked with cholesterol. The debate of the etiology of this condition is centered on whether this begins in the head or the heart. Regardless of the answer, the heart is the damaged target organ.

THE HEART IN RELIGION

To even begin to understand the heart's influence on our society and in our cultures, we can study the heart as a symbol and the organ's philosophical underpinnings. In this section I hope to show how the heart is woven into the roots of religious philosophy and prayers, with an emphasis on prayers.

The heart's influence is wide-ranging and leads through many doorways into other rooms of history, where many crucial contributions to our medical and emotional evolutions can also be found. I will, however, do my best to remember this essay is about the heart and not get sidetracked by the many other fascinating aspects of the civilizations I am looking into.

I begin this chapter with the seventeenth-century French mathematician, scientist, and philosopher Blaise Pascal, who was raised in a conventional Catholic family that came under the influence of Jansenism, a rigorous Catholic movement in France, influenced by Calvin's Protestantism and ultimately condemned by the Church as heretical. Jansenism held that God's grace was only attributable to God, thus negating human depravity in an effort to earn or achieve a spiritual state of grace. Out of this fraught background grew Pascal's insight, captured in his famous quote: "Le coeur a ses raisons que la raison ne connaît point"—*The heart has its reasons, which reason knows nothing of.* He reasoned there are three levels of knowledge: the body, comprised of the senses; mind, or reason; and heart, or faith. Each is valid in its own way.

When we think of liturgical traditions, we may first think of the Hebrew bible and all it has passed down to us throughout our history, but we need to probe archaic religions.

The cuneiform tablets that have survived from city-states like Uruk and Babylon are primarily for business accounting and contain no decipherable narratives except for the saga of Gilgamesh. Fragments of prayers, however, have been found, at least one of which references the heart:

> What seems good to oneself is a crime before the god.
> What to one's heart seems bad, is good before one's god.

Already we can see that these ancient civilizations have begun to center the heart as a repository of human feeling, even as the mystery of how the gods may be ordering the world is proclaimed.

Ancient Egypt gives us more to work with as regards the heart. The heart is a central figure in ancient Egyptian religion and is itself a symptom of the changed relation between god, king—in Egypt called pharaoh—and human citizens. This basic concept of the pharaoh as a conduit to god is linked to the First, Middle, and Old Kingdoms and encompasses a span of two to three thousand years. Over the centuries, however, the relationship between god and pharaoh was altered. In the end, there is no mention of the individual's heart, but there is an acknowledgment that the heart of the king thinks and plans for all, much as an all-seeing god does.

The religious quantum leap for Israel occurred when the relationship of God and the Children of Israel became a covenant between God and his worshippers, in contrast to an Egyptian hierarchy with a king as an intermediary between a god and the king's people, who were overseen as vassals.

For the prophet Jeremiah, one key word is heart, in Hebrew (*lev*):

> Now hear this, O people foolish and without heart, who
> have eyes but do not see.

Subsequent, less literal, translations, as well as the King James version of the book of Jeremiah interpret "without heart" as "without understanding," a revision of the text which only serves to emphasize the ancient roots of our linking the heart—fundamentally the organ circulating blood and oxygen throughout our body—to our feelings and emotional experience of ourselves and the world around us.

The Psalmist too depends upon the audience knowing that the heart is the source of logic, emotion, and equanimity: "Wine makes empty the heart and bread nourishes the heart." Already the physical and metaphoric treatments of the heart are being united, as the speaker of this song acknowledges the physical effects of alcohol and solid sustenance on not just the body, but the emotions of those who are sadly drinking and happily eating.

Where do we go from this introduction to the heart?

As I mentioned before, the Hebrew for heart is *lev*, but frequently, the version used is *levou*, a pluralized form, indicating more than one heart, which might call to mind the two atria and two ventricles. When the heart is discussed as the abode of the soul the term is *rooach*. Despite that other plural form, the rabbis and prophets in biblical passages about the heart regard the heart as the seat of the intellect, emotion, and understanding, not as the circulatory pump.

Some passages imply the heart and stomach are the same organ. In Genesis 18:5, Abraham welcomes the strangers with offers of feeding the strangers "bread to the heart." There is much potential discussion about the connection of the gastrointestinal tract and the heart through the vagus nerve which supplies both systems, as we now know. This is not the place to revise the several contemporary Hebrew terms for heart in its relation to various gastrointestinal and emotional states. What is important to remember is the symbolic sense of *lev*, now and in the past, indicating the heart is regarded as the seat of emotion and intelligence.

To end this discussion of the heart in the Hebrew liturgical tradition, the famous sixteenth-century Code of Jewish Law by Joseph Caro should be addressed here. According to the framework his scholarship established, the heart is not necessary or needed. The exemplifying story goes as follows: If a victim is severely injured and not expected to live, the rescuer must expose the nose and examine the victim carefully for any signs of breathing. If there is no evidence of breath from the nose, the person is dead under the code of Jewish law. Maimonides, the twelfth-century philosopher, would agree with this approach and conclusion. Neither Maimonides nor Caro requires an examination of the heart through feeling a pulse or hearing or feeling a heartbeat when determining life. Cessation of respiration is the determining physical sign of death.

The Hebrew Bible does include vague descriptions of cardiac anatomy. These are discussed further in the Talmud and Mishnah by rabbis and learned teachers commenting on the original texts. However, the cardiac anatomy is primitive, citing two chambers of the heart—the right and left ventricles—and this knowledge is clearly obtained from ritual slaughter of animals, rather than from direct human cardiac examination or dissection.

But the Judeo-Christian traditions are not the only liturgical and philosophical traditions in our histories. To get the broadest view of the ways humanity has ascribed meaning to the heart beyond its mechanical and physical functions, we must also look beyond the Mediterranean and its surrounding neighbors.

When we look at the influence of China, two physicians are remarkable. The first is Mencius—in Chinese, Mengzi—one of two Chinese thinkers whose reach and influence have been so broad that their names have long since been Latinized by Europeans; the other is Confucius.

Mencius lived a century after Confucius in the fourth century BCE. Mencius is famous for arguing that human nature is good. Mencius assumes human nature has the potentiality to develop virtue—he is a moralist. Mencius declares, "No man is devoid of a heart sensitive to the suffering of others." The heart (*xin*) is a key term in his moral philosophy, as it was also in earlier Chinese work such as the Guanzi, a foundational collection of philosophical, medical, and administrative essays from pre–Common Era China. Under this approach, vital energy (*qi*) is the source of moral action of the learned. Such extraordinary qi is born of accumulated rightness which "is set in the heart." The heart is the source of moral feelings.

Xunzi, a philosopher contemporary with Mencius, rejects Mencius's idea that human nature is good. His idea of the heart is indebted to the fact that it does not have a moral intuition. He sets up a paradoxical exercise to explain his understanding of the heart's absence of morality, asking: How does man know the way? His answer: By the heart. But then he asks: How does the heart know? Which returns us to the question of how man knows. This very complex circuitous argument that follows has been difficult for both Chinese and Western philosophers to unravel. So, I will leave Xunzi's argument here, noting that the question of how the heart and mind understand each other remains unanswered for Xunzi.

Finally, let us look at the roots of Islamic medicine as it pertains to the heart. Please remember, Islamic history is long and wide-ranging—this discussion is only concerning the legacy of the Prophet Muhammad's word on especially the heart.

In the case of Islam the revelation is the Quran, while the recipient of that revelation is the Prophet Muhammad. It is in the light of the prophetic function in Islam that the medicine of the prophet must be understood. Traditional Islamic medicine functioned in a world in which spirit, soul, and body reigned in unity. The sickness of the heart concerns more than mechanical function; the center of the human microcosmos is also the site, or the locus, of the spirit and soul. These aspects of the heart are concerned with the reality of God.

Medicine of the heart is entrusted to the messengers, who are the prophets Muslims believe are sent by God, to serve as examples of ideal human behavior. Tranquility of the heart is obtained through sudden insight of the Lord and Creator and his attributes. Only then can true health be found. The health of the heart can be achieved only by following the messengers. As Muhammad proclaims in the Quran, "The heart was created for the knowledge and love of its Creator, acknowledge His Oneness; delight in Him; remember Him."

We can see from these glimpses into ancient annals from religious and philosophical traditions that our myriad cultures have, through hundreds of years, imbued the heart with a power and meaning beyond its physical properties alone. Even when overlooking its crucial role in keeping us alive, as Maimonides did, our traditions still grant the heart a symbolic power to be empty, to be sated, to keep our souls safe or to tempt them to go against the gods themselves.

These roots may seem distant and isolated, but the heart's symbolic influence permeates our world, and the historic influence of Byzantine art, religion, and medicine can be seen even today.

In my travels, I have been several times to Venice and often visited its Accademia dell'Arte Museum. This museum, prior to Napoleon's conquest of Italy in 1804, was the Church of the Carità, dating from the thirteenth century. The present building was rebuilt in 1441 and 1452, while still a religious institution, under the Augustinians. The museum also includes the adjoining building of the original cloister and school. When you enter the museum, the staircases on the right and left sides contain the life-size statues of Faith and Charity by G. M. Morlaitor. One statue holds a flaming heart and the other cradles a sculpted heart held in her hand. These each represent the Sacred Heart of Jesus—this prominent celebration of Jesus in the Catholic Church, centered on the veneration of Jesus's physical heart as a representation of Jesus's love and sacrifice, began to be practiced in the tenth century and increased throughout the Middle Ages and the Renaissance.

Ironically the Catholic cult of the Sacred Heart of Jesus flourished contemporaneously with William Harvey's *De Motu Cordis* (1628), the first accurate description of the circulation of the blood.

Ah Love! Could thou and I with fate conspire
To grasp this sorry Scheme of Things entire,
Would we not shatter it to bits—and then
Re-mould it nearer to the Heart's Desire!

—Omar Khayyam
Perisan poet, 1048–1131

~~

The Blind Men and The Elephant

The beast, and each, by feeling trunk or limb,
Strove to acquire an image clear of him.
Thus each conceived a visionary whole,
And to the phantom clung with heart and soul.

—Rumi (Jalāl ad-Dīn Muḥammad Balkhī)
Persian poet, 1207–1273

~~

The perfume of thy curls across my cheek.
A dart from thy bent brows has wounded me—
Ah, come! My heart still waiteth helplessly.

—Hafiz
(Khāwje Shams-od-Dīn Moḥammad Ḥāfeẓ-e Shīrāzī)
Persian poet, d. 1390

~~

A new heart will I give you,
A new spirit within you.
I will remove the heart of stone from
your flesh and give you a heart
that feels.
—*The New Union Prayer Book for the Days of Atonement*
Yom Kipper Morning Service

EGYPT

Medicine is a well-documented aspect of ancient Egyptian life. The Egyptians were the first people to get close to developing a medical understanding of the physical heart, to link the heart's function to signs of health or disease. But even so, they were hindered by the importance of the symbolic heart to their understanding of the world and an individual's passage through it.

The ancient Egyptian hieroglyph for the heart, *ib*, goes through several iterations over the many centuries of written records. This early hieroglyph begins as an image of an ox heart. Ib represents the metaphysical entity ancient Egyptians ascribed to the heart, and this concept embodies thought, intelligence, memory, wisdom, bravery, sadness, and love. The hieroglyph of the heart was first drawn with vessels attached during the archaic period (3168–2705 BCE) in the first and second dynasties. After the third dynasty the symbol was modified to resemble a heart-shaped jar, and persisted as such throughout the third through the sixth dynasties (Old Kingdom, 2705–2260 BCE).

The anatomical heart was referred to by a different word, *haty*, and Egyptians worked to understand the object's physical purpose. Several medical papyri have been found that provide a picture of what the Egyptians called "the necessary art." Egyptian physicians were quite adept in the treatment of injuries, as revealed in the Edwin Smith Surgical Papyrus, an early and surprisingly in-depth medical text dating from the second century BCE, which outlines various diagnoses and treatments of different types of injuries. If an illness was of unknown etiology, however, then physicians attributed the distemper to magic, and religion was invoked in the subsequent cures.

Because of this intimacy between medicine and religion at this time, prominent physicians could also be found in the roles of priests presiding in religious temples. In ancient Egypt, as in many places, man received medical knowledge through the gods. The earliest doctors were magicians.

The study of ancient Egyptian science and medicine has become a voluminous task, due to the many insights and the many written records the Egyptians left. For our purposes, I will concentrate my review on their understanding of the heart in its dual nature.

Egyptian rational medicine was the best in the world in and around 2200 to 1500 BCE. Egyptian doctors were sent to the courts of kings throughout the Middle East, with their knowledge and approaches ultimately affecting Greek, Arabic, and medieval medicine.

The Ebers Papyrus, dating from the same era as the Smith Surgical Papyrus, contains a section that deals specifically with the heart and its vessels. This section proclaims its import in its title: "The beginning of the seizing of the physician. To know the movements of the heart and to know the heart." Thanks to this and other records, we know Egyptian doctors recognized the relationship of the heart to the pulse but had no idea of the method of circulation. They could feel the pulse by putting the finger on a neck, hand, arm, or leg.

Egyptian medicine also recognized the heart is the center of the vascular system and the vessels attach to it from the organ of the body. In the Ebers Papyrus, Pharoh Usaphis says, "Man hath twelve vessels proceeding from his heart which extend to his body and limbs; two vessels go to each leg and to each arm; two vessels to the front and back of the head; two branches go to the eyes; two to the nose, two vessels to the right ear"—literally, *the breath of life goes through them*—and two are described as connecting to the left ear and through them passes the breath of death, according to the papyrus.

Remember, the Egyptians considered the heart a well—not a pump. In many ways, their model was based on their immediate environment. Water was distributed in Egypt through a vast network of canals emanating from the Nile River. This explains their concept of the heart as a source, rather than a circulatory instrument, and of the vessels emanating from it as streams flowing away from it. Besides carrying blood, the vessels were said to carry air, urine, feces, sperm, and tears.

They realized the pulses that they could feel and measure emanated from the heart, but any deeper understanding of the circulatory process was stymied by the immense gravitational pull of the seminal concept of the heart's symbolic role. The physicians' manual outlines how, when the heart is sad, the pulse is weak and the vessels are filled with air and water—not blood. They knew that fever increased the pulse rate, and they came close to understanding the interdependence of the pulmonary and circulatory systems. They thought that breathing moved the air from the nose to the heart and intestine, to then be expelled via the anus. Though the oxygen in the air we breathe does find its way to the heart, the process is largely different from what the ancient Egyptians envisioned.

Most importantly to the Egyptians, and to us as their infinitely influenced heirs, the heart is the seat of consciousness and character. For the Egyptians the home of consciousness was located not in the brain but in the heart, which was for them the controlling force within the body. The heart was where the thought processes began, to be then uttered through the mouth, the organ they believed most intimately connected to the heart's metaphysical work.

This metaphysical work or substance was central to their burial rituals and their beliefs of the afterlife. Egyptian burial practice removed many of the body's important organs to prepare for embalming—liver, lungs, intestines, and stomach were all placed in separate canopic jars as part of the preparations for the afterlife. But the heart was never removed, because it was far too important. Instead, the embalmer would often put inside the chest, next to the heart or the chest wall, a carved stone scarab engraved with messages to the deceased. A scarab is carved in the shape of a beetle, the symbol of eternal life. The scarab beetle, or dung beetle, was universally worshipped by the Egyptians. The beetles laid their eggs in dung balls fashioned through rolling scat, which then underwent a miraculous rebirth and became a symbol of regeneration. The Egyptian heart scarab was also used as an amulet and as jewelry, as protection and as a reminder of the symbolic meaning and importance of this central organ.

The Egyptian god Ptah, whose heart and tongue, with his intentions and breath, brought the gods themselves into being, presides over the heart and tongue. But Anubis is the god who traditionally weighs the heart in the afterlife, thus determining whether the newly deceased was a good or bad person. Sight, hearing, and breathing all report to the heart and then the tongue that then repeats what the heart has derived using the balance scale.

The Book of the Dead shows this crucial narrative of the afterlife: the heart resting on one balance pan, and a feather—the emblem of Maat, the goddess of truth—on the other. If the deceased has led a moral life the two pans are level. To be able to be judged truly in the next world, one must have the heart still in the body, ready and waiting to reveal all the truth of the person's decisions, deeds, thoughts, and speech. Without the heart, one cannot progress into the afterlife.

The Book of the Dead is replete with many spells that reflect the centrality of the heart in Egyptian life and thought. The spell for going out in the day expresses the common awareness of both the emotional and physical importance of the heart to the conduct of life: "May I have power in my heart, arms and legs." To combat helpless feelings, there is a spell to take control of one's environment and claim power for one's heart. And along with the scarab amulets, there is a spell for not permitting a heart to be taken from the body in the realm of the dead.

Finally, there are a variety of fragments of hieroglyphic writing from the many centuries of ancient Egyptian culture and thought. Much of this writing, in poetry and song, portrays the heart in metaphors and images that are still familiar to us as modern souls, so many centuries from when they were written and half a world away from where they were found.

How lovely is your sister, the darling of your heart.

I have abandoned my brother—then I remember your love—my heart within stands still.

My heart has a portion of yours, I do its will for you when I am in your arms.

My brother, my loved one, my heart chases after your love and all that has been fashioned by you.

Now must I depart from the brother and as I long for your love, my heart stands still inside me.

As my sole concern I have set the love of my brother; for him my heart will not keep silent.

My heart it was that urged me to do my duty in accordance with its instructions.

I was not drunken. My heart was not forgetful. I was not negligent in my actions. My heart it was that raised my station.

A brave heart in situation of wretchedness is a companion for its lord.

Make yourself heavy in your heart, make your heart steadfast. Don't steer with your tongue.

All divine speech originated from that which was thought up by the heart and commanded by the tongue.
                              —Ancient Egyptian fragments

MESOPOTAMIA

My challenge in this chapter is to navigate the lands around and between the two rivers, the Tigris and the Euphrates. Here the first cities were established in the fourth, third, second, and first millennia BCE during the Babylonian, Assyrian, and Persian Empires. This vast area roughly encompasses the contemporary nations of Syria, Iran, and Iraq. The biblical regions of Israel, Jordan, and Lebanon overlap this history, but do not directly affect this overview. Over the centuries of countless wars, the boundary lines of kingdoms and city-states were continuously altered.

Despite their ancient roots, the written records of civilizations that flourished in this area show people who worked hard on survival but were only able to rigorously explore questions of medicinal cause and effect much later than the Egyptians, who had already begun writing the surgical and analytical treatises that have come down to us. Unlike the Egyptians, the people of Mesopotamia had strict prohibitions against human dissection, so had no way of increasing their knowledge of the physical function of the heart beyond what they could learn from a patient's symptoms, or from the animals they were allowed to slaughter and examine. As a result, they made many assumptions about the human heart's shape and function from their analyses of sheep hearts.

For these civilizations, disease was supernatural in origin and due to the activity of the unseen spirits of ghosts and demons inhabiting the body of the sufferer. Demonic possession of the diseased person was often assumed to be induced by a deity and, perhaps, a human sorcerer. Any possible cure depended upon the dislodgment of the evil presence by a higher divine power. Therefore, treatment of disease was primarily a religious matter under the direction and supervision of priests.

Babylonian medicine specifically ascribed the ultimate cause of diseases or illnesses to divine punishment, and was not divorced from magic. Babylonians were fond of lists, leaving many records which include not just rosters of medical herbal remedies but also catalogs of parts of the body. According to their records, they appear to have never advanced much from the original concepts they outlined for themselves. They often just recopied documents over the centuries without adding new knowledge or information to the records, even as these records accrued.

The Akkadians, however, had detailed words for the heart. This knowledge, however, was obtained from their examinations of sheep hearts, and so we must remember that these words and concepts were applied to a human heart as if the anatomy were exactly the same:

> Rear part of the heart: Warkat libbim
> Lower part of the heart: Elinu libbim
> Joint part of the heart: Kisir libbim
> Thick part of the heart: Kubur libbim
> Pericardium: Saman libbim
> Fortress of the heart: Dur libbim
> Apex of the heart: Res libbim

While the overwhelming belief in the religious and magical connections of illness and cures hampered their ability to outline direct medical treatments for physical systems, the Mesopotamian cultures, like that of the Egyptians, did recognize the pulse as a key aspect of life and health. The rhythm of the pulse was recognized to shift and change in harmony with symptoms such as a discoloration of skin and the lighter or darker color of urine.

Nothing else comes down to us about the physiology and disorders of the heart from the Mesopotamian priests or doctors. Enter the poets.

Three millennia ago, female goddess-healers were these societies' most worshipped healers, predating women's medical healing skills in our contemporary society. The goddess Gula is perhaps the one that was most widespread.

Archaeologists digging in Iraq first reported to the public in 1990 the uncovering of the ruins of a huge temple—larger than a football field—to the Babylonian goddess of healing and patron of physicians, Gula. Gula as the word and the name itself is translated as *great*. The site is sixty miles southeast of Baghdad and dates to between 1600 BCE and 1200 BCE. Dog figurines are found at this site, firmly establishing Gula's identity and indicating the use of the site; several other sites throughout Mesopotamia have been also identified with Gula because they include dog burials and clay dog votive offerings. Her worship as a healing goddess may have started in a single area, but thanks to these sites we know that it spread and was well-established throughout this region.

Across ancient Mesopotamian history and cultures, Gula appears in different guises, but always identified with a dog. The symbolic link of dogs and healers may be seen to start here, perhaps based in the simple observation of domesticated dogs licking their wounds and associating that cleansing action with the healing process. The depth of this association may start with Gula, and it certainly spread with her temples and worship— the renowned Greek physician Aesculapius one thousand years later has a similar association with dogs.

Gula is a goddess of healing. She helps breathe life into mankind after the Great Flood. She is described as a great physician of "the black-headed people," referring to the Sumerians. Gula is also the ancient name for the Earth Mother Goddess, who was consort of Ninurta, a Mesopotamian god who was the patron of herbs, healing, and life. Though these attributes and powers deal with the physical level of the body, and thus, implicitly, the heart itself, the spiritual aspect of the heart and all it conveys retains its primacy under Gula and throughout the region. This intense connection of the heart to concepts of emotion and intellect arguably obscured the other, physical, connections that might have been made between the heart and its connection to the body's physical health. Even the priestesses of Gula who worked with physically ill people might not have been able to see beyond the mysticism, especially because any empirical examinations through human dissection were strictly forbidden.

We know, from fragments of prayers, how Gula was appreciated. One prayer of thanks reads, "May the sages apply the bandages! You, Gula, have brought about health and healing." This text recognizes the belief that all medical procedures were directed by the will of the deity.

Mesopotamia was also home to the poet Enheduanna, whose writings are among the oldest recorded poems. Enheduanna was a Sumerian poet, who wrote in 2200 BCE (1,700 years before Sappho, 1,100 years before Homer) and who is the earliest known poet whose name has been recognized. She lived in the Sumerian city of Ur, in modern Iraq.

Her poem *Inanna, Lady of Largest Heart* has been pieced together from many fragments and, though fragmented, runs to over four thousand lines.

Her writings reveal the centrality of the heart's role in Mesopotamian culture. Much as the Egyptians thought of the heart as the center of feeling, thought, and emotion, Enheduanna too treats the heart as the repository of emotion. For her, as for Mesopotamian culture of this time, the symbolic or emotional heart has attained primacy over any known physical aspects. She speaks of a "cruel heart"; one character "gladdens her heart"; the poem describes "soft whispers in her heart."

Enheduanna is the poet whose name has been preserved over these many centuries, but other fragments of poems and prayers, without authors attached, are also part of our historic record.

Fragments of Babylonian poetry reveal how the heart was a focus of thought and emotion—anxiety as expressed by how the poets' hearts feel, worries about lovers' desires, and their hopeful returns are but a few examples of the importance that Babylonians ascribed to the metaphysical heart.

Ugaritic narrative poems come from the ancient city of Ugarit, lying a half mile inland from the Syrian coast, opposite the eastern tip of Cyprus. They originate from approximately 1350 BCE and include the only ancient records of poetry and narrative outside of the Hebrew bible in this coastal region. The Ugaritic texts were written and recorded at a more distant site from the Tigris-Euphrates valley than the other texts I reference here. Yet they too signal the primacy of the metaphysical heart as a seat of emotion and its significance to their concept of themselves and those around them.

All of these cultures gave to their symbolic hearts abstract qualities and urgency that are familiar to us, even today—love, sorrow, fear, desire, and anger are all represented and symbolized by their references to the heart.

Grind my knees in your neck
till tears wet your face
sorrow grips your heart.

— Enheduanna

My god has forsaken me and disappeared
My goddess has failed me
The king, the flesh of the gods, the sun of his people
His heart is enraged with life even not be appeased.

I want my hearts' love to come in.
        dragon of AN
I will place my hand in his hand.
                        touch   heart to his heart

You ask for the mountain
        want the heart of it—he says this to her
        The Queen
        Ask for Mount Ebih
        want the heart of it he says to her

—Babylonian fragments

They rejoin exceedingly
Their heart rejoices

Like the heart of cow for the calf
        ewe for her lamb
So is the heart of ANAT for Baal

El laughs in his heart
Quivers in his liver

—Ugaritic fragments

GREEK AND ROMAN MEDICINE

Ancient Greek and Roman approaches to medicine are intimately interwoven, as were their cultures. Greece, however, being the earlier marriage of political and cultural power, provided the material for Rome, as it rose to prominence, to use or disregard as its citizenry, and its leaders, preferred.

The history of how the early Greeks understood the human heart centers around Greek mythology. The well-known Orphic, Promethean, and Dionysian myths are about death, rebirth, and regeneration, and they each implicitly treat the heart as the center of the flesh. As with neighboring cultures and religions, the heart is considered, for the ancient and the classical Greeks, to be the principal source of life.

This unique status of the human heart was not simply limited to Greek myths but reverberated throughout the entire culture. The fourth-century Greek philosopher Aristotle, in *De Moto Animalium*, writes the heart is not only the origin and center of life but is the guiding metaphor for the structure of the city-state, or polis. Aristotle says that the heart is devoted to life in general, and this understanding is central to much of his analysis of both the philosophical and natural worlds. Due to Aristotle's immense influence, and his many works that have been preserved for us, this heart-centric principle dominated scientific thought through the centuries.

When contemplating the studying of Greek medicine as archaeologists and historians, we usually use Hippocrates as the starting point. However, if a thorough understanding of the roots of Greek cardiology is the goal, the student must begin with Empedocles (c. 490–430 BCE), who lived and worked just before Hippocrates, in the fifth century BCE. Sadly, much of what this remarkable man has written is lost. What we do know is that his works influenced philosophers, theologians, and biologists of his time and after. Empedocles's view of the heart and its importance to the intellect is expressed in one of the remaining fragments of his work:

> In the blood-streams, back-leaping into it,
> The heart is nourished, where prevails the power
> That men call thought; for, lo, the blood that stirs
> About the heart is man's controlling thought.

Empedocles also describes the four elements of fire, air, earth, and water, linking them to hot, cold, dry, and wet states, all of which needed to be variously balanced or controlled for a healthy body and mind. He claimed that blood contained a balance of all four elements, and he asserted that human thought existed in the blood surrounding the heart. Empedocles's insights about the importance of blood and the beating heart were still bound up with other concepts that earlier groups, including the Egyptians and the Mesopotamians, had also made about the physical heart's control over a person's thoughts and feelings. And even as Empedocles worked to outline the way the heart could indeed influence physical and mental health, the balance of the eight elements remained a central component of his analysis of the body's mechanical functions.

Scholars who have studied Hippocrates's collected writings, the *Corpus Hippocraticum*, consider the section on the heart to reflect Empedocles's insights and understandings of how the blood and the heart worked. Empedocles may even have given this section to Hippocrates or, perhaps, Hippocrates repeated it wholesale from Empedocles's groundbreaking work, with or without Empedocles's blessing—we may never know.

Despite the Greeks' academic primacy throughout these centuries, the center of academic learning did not remain for long in their original Hellenic lands. Aristotle's most famous student was, ultimately, Alexander the Great, who conquered vast lands across the Mediterranean and into Mesopotamia, Anatolia, and India to create an empire that was world-encompassing for those who were in it. Alexander founded Alexandria in Egypt as the center of his growing empire, and it remained a central and powerful city after the breakup of his lands in the wake of his death. Alexandria remained the capital city after the division of Alexander's empire, when Egypt was successfully inherited by Ptolomy I, and within a generation or two it cemented its enduring status as the most important academic and medical center in the Ancient Near East. The Library at Alexandria, a pet project of Ptolomy's heirs, became both a crucial reference collection and a wondrous attraction for anyone interested in furthering not just their own knowledge but knowledge for all to share.

The Library, one assumes, is what drew two important Greek medical scholars to Alexandria in the third century BCE—Herophilus and Erasistratus. Though no complete work by either man survives for us to study as a primary source, the second-century Greek medical doctor Galen—who finished his life as a Roman citizen—allows us a window into the anatomic and physiologic work of these two Greek physicians through his own, later, writings.

Herophilus posited that the brain be understood as the center of the central nervous system and the basis of the intellect. As we recall, Aristotle gave this role to the heart. Herophilus placed a great deal of emphasis on empirical study and observation, and he dissected live prisoners and cadavers. These observations led him to refute Aristotle's assertions, and instead to argue for the brain's importance to physiological understanding. Like the Egyptians, he understood the importance of the pulse, and he taught that the beat of the heart caused the pulse in the wall of the artery. The pulse was counted by a water clock he set up to mimic the ideal pulse rate for patients of various ages. He measured the pulse with this specially calibrated water clock, and he spoke of the rhythm of music in his study of the pulse.

Erasistratus, another student of medicine who made his way to Alexandria a few years after Herophilus, studied the heart valves. He saw the heart as a pump, but erroneously deduced that the blood was made in the liver. In his schema, the heart and arteries carried *pneuma*, or breath, and veins carried blood, each from the heart to the body parts through their own pathways.

He taught the pneuma flowed in the arteries and mixed with blood in the heart. He also asserted that veins supplied, through capillary beds, blood into the arteries—a route that is the reverse of the true path of circulatory flow.

Erasistratus envisioned the heart as a one-way pump, but carried the concept of circulation no further. The concept of the pump, however, was revolutionary. At the time of Aristotle and Hippocrates the Greek language did not contain a word for *pump*, and Erasistratus appears to be the first to have so envisioned it as a concept in physiology.

While these Greek philosophers and natural historians were wrestling with the concepts of humors and attempting to comprehend how the heart and the blood actually interact, Rome, and thus Roman medicine, had not yet grown into the more organized Roman Empire we usually envision at this time.

Rome was an Etruscan city in the seventh and sixth centuries BCE. The Etruscans from about 800 BCE inhabited Italy from the Tiber River in the south to the Po River in the north. The Etruscans absorbed Greek philosophy and thought, and the Greeks ultimately influenced the Roman idea that the primitive *numina*—divine powers or spirits which presided locally or were believed to inhabit a particular object—were fused with a deity with human form that combined early Greek and Etruscan beliefs.

Many ceramic Etruscan votives representing diseased or injured parts of the body have been found in the ruins of Etruscan temples, left there in the hope of a cure. A few represent very stylized interval viscera, including the heart. These were used to ask for relief from disease, as part of this culture's magical approach to the management of illness.

Magical treatment was common for the Etruscans, as seen through this votive use, and for the early Romans. Though cures based outright in religious rituals or magical beliefs were rarer, exhibiting a kind of rationality which was characteristic of early Roman medicine.

The sources that have survived concern themselves with only remedies, for the most part. Diagnoses and prognoses were not taken into serious consideration. Throughout the Etruscan period and into the early stages of Roman development, religious and magical outlooks determined healing. The Romans felt the gods were supreme lords and all events were directed by their wisdom and divine power and intervention.

The Romans adapted and frequently employed Etruscan augury and divination to ward off disease throughout all levels of society. Etruscan priests conducted rites to discern the will of the gods. Over the centuries the Etruscan way of life reluctantly gave way to a more specifically Roman one, as Rome gradually accepted and adopted Greek medicine, adding the Greek knowledge of and approach to physiology to their practice of medicine.

Early Roman medical texts were first compiled by Cato the Elder, who lived from 239 to 149 BCE. He saw Greek influence as a threat to Roman tradition. Cato was not a physician, but rather a historian who was intent on preserving Roman practice without any changes from foreign cultures. His writings recommend treatments that mix magical incantations with various animal and vegetable remedies. His folk medicine relies remarkably heavily on the use of cabbage.

Pliny the Elder, who followed Cato two centuries later, was another encyclopedist who worked to preserve Roman cultural traditions free from Greek influence. This thread of Roman thinkers refusing to acknowledge contributing insights from other cultures prevented Roman medicine from embracing the advances obtainable through empirical observation of anatomy and surgery.

Thus ancient Roman medicine made no original contribution to the heart and vascular system, and leaned on Etruscan and Greek medical theory for the practice of medicine.

Galen, the famous Greek physician and natural scientist who in 169 CE was called to Rome to be physician to the Roman emperor Marcus Aurelius, exemplifies the apex of Greek medicine and how adeptly Greek knowledge became integral to the functioning of the Roman Empire. Galen of Pergamum was born in 129 CE, and as a young man he studied medicine in Pergamum, located in the heart of Greek territory, and in Alexandria in Egypt. His early medical career was in Pergamum as a physician to gladiators. In this role he learned anatomy and surgery.

Galen produced an enormous corpus of writings, including eighteen books on the pulse alone. His observation of the heart and blood vessels was complex and relied on the work of earlier Greek physicians, including Herophilus and Hippocrates. He was a medical doctor who began as a natural scientist, embraced experimentation and new medical knowledge, and ended his life in Rome as a theologian. His claim "All created by God has a purpose" exemplifies his journey from empiricism through philosophy to, finally, theology.

Because of his breadth of knowledge and his wealth of writings, his influence extended for centuries throughout what would become Europe and the Middle East. His insistence that blood passed through tiny holes in the wall between the ventricles froze the knowledge of the circulation for

1,400 years—until William Harvey's 1628 treatise that accurately traced the movement of blood from the heart to the lungs and back again before circulating throughout the body.

Despite that misleading thesis of a permeable membrane in the heart, Galen did understand and prove that the arteries contained not breath but blood. He noted the parts of the heart, though he didn't understand their functions precisely, and he described how the right auricle—the right atrium—outlived the rest of the heart, being the last part to stop contracting when life was over.

Galen assigned importance to the parts of the body by their placement as much as their function, noting that the liver was the lowest fundamental member of the body, with the heart being the fundamental member of the middle, and the brain of the upper. He did agree with Aristotle that the pneuma, or spirit, was important to these organs, and each fundamental member was described by Galen as being dominated by a special pneuma. The heart pneuma, *zotikon*, was, for Galen and his fellow practitioners, transported in the veins to be mixed with air inside the heart, producing the blood for the body.

In summary, despite the many things they observed and studied about the heart and the vascular system, the ancient Greeks, and then the Romans, knew little about cardiac physiology. One problem for modern scholars of ancient Greek medicine that prevents a clear picture of the limits of Greek medical knowledge is the double meaning of the word *kardia*. In classical Greek, this word translates as both the heart and the mouth of the esophagus.

Nor is this inquiry made any simpler by the various theories of the seat of consciousness and the center of the nervous system. Aristotle held the center of the nervous system was the heart, sometimes including the adjacent diaphragm muscles, and he assumed that all mental conditions arose from this area. On the other hand, there is evidence that there were other Greek and Roman thinkers who regarded the brain as the seat of consciousness and associated the heart, lungs, and stomach with conditions of humoral imbalance.

Both Aristotle's and Galen's vast amount of writings, however, are the main works of medicine, physiology, and natural science that have been preserved over the centuries. As writings that have remained accessible and have endured, they have been more influential across time and are our only understanding of how the Greeks and Romans best understood the physiological importance of the heart.

What we can see from Greek and Roman writings overall is that Greek and Roman medical knowledge was not entirely scientific. Both cultures were more influenced by religion and philosophy and not what we would consider modern scientific inquiry, which would focus on the physiologic connections of the body over the philosophical concerns of the humors and how they should balance. Galen, despite his reliance on empirical observation throughout his surgical career, ended up a philosopher and a poet, searching through his medical experience not only for a path to health but for a purpose and meaning to life in a world created by a greater force than humanity itself.

Thus, we can see that Aristotle's focus on the heart as a physical and emotional center of the body reflects humanity's overarching predilection to treat the heart as the source of feeling—from love to despair.

Sappho, the most creative poet in the history of the Western world, wrote in the sixth century BCE, over a century before Aristotle began theorizing about the humors inhabiting our hearts. Fragments of her work have survived, and many of these exemplify her impulse to grapple with her feelings through the concept of the heart.

Sappho's heart is hopeful, is shaken by love, and is set aflame by the sight of her lover. Sappho—like Aristotle and, even later, Galen— understands the heart as key to human life. Instead of linking it physically to health or the pulse, however, Sappho reveals how fragile it can feel, as a symbol, and how the emotions of love and fear and hope can impact the very life in our chest as extremely as Galen's gladiators would later be stricken by the physical blows of their combatants.

For the Romans and the Greeks, the heart is key to human life on both the physical and metaphysical levels, and the importance of both levels together made it impossible for them to see clearly the physical cardiology structures that our medical knowledge now relies on at the cellular level. We continue to be influenced by their beliefs—both the accurate and the misleading—that the heart is the core of one's being, and that the heart is where our existence is found.

What my heart most hopes will
happen, make happen; you yourself
join forces on my side!

As a whirlwind
swoops on an oak
Love shakes my heart

That hayseed in her hair—
such finery—has put
a torch to your heart

Gold is God's child
neither worms nor
moths eat gold; it
is much stronger
than a man's heart

—Sappho, fragments

If the coming of Spring shivers
the dancing leaves, or some green lizard
twitches a bramble,
his knees and heart quake

~~

Now I would change
those acid lines for sweet, if only (since I take
back all my taunts) you'll be my friend
and give me back my heart

~~

If some untimely blow should take you
the half of my heart, ah, why should I linger

— Horace

THE MEDIEVAL HEART

Western society's interpretation and understanding of the heart during the medieval period, from the eleventh to the fifteenth centuries CE, is difficult to embrace. There are no systematic scientific explorations of the heart by physicians during that time. Philosophers of the era seemed to rely primarily on the ancient Greek philosophers, especially Aristotle.

Because of this reliance on Aristotle and, where applicable, Galen for their knowledge of the heart's function, and because of the general prohibition against anatomical dissection, the Western European medieval tradition does not add any new knowledge of the heart's physiological functions. Medieval thinkers, especially philosophers and poets, instead developed an expressive language of the heart. The heart was central to medieval poetry and music, as well as to the religious concepts of faith and God as understood by the Catholic Church, the primary religious institution of Western Europe during this period.

Modern scholar Eric Jager's elaborate "The Scriptorium of the Heart," in his *The Book of the Heart*, sets the stage for medieval treatments about the heart. This chapter details how scholastic and monastic writings not only constructed books about the heart, but also built an understanding of the heart itself as a book. Jager draws parallels between the physical writings of faith and the actions of faith as they worked in the body and in the heart as the central component of the body. During the Middle Ages these intellectual exercises are central to the monastic tradition. As monastic influence begins to permeate all levels of medieval life, the heart becomes a vessel for the experience of faith as well as love—these two pathways of romantic love and religious faith become increasingly tied together as they share the heart as their most important home in the physical and conceptual body.

As early as the tenth century CE, the Jewish physician and poet Moses Ben Abraham Dar'ī said the heart was an alert and active romantic force. We can see that this concentration on the heart as a center of emotional life is not, during this period, confined to Catholic influences, and that it extends across all classes and religions in this society.

Heather Webb in her 2010 monograph, *The Medieval Heart*, points out we speak of the heart according to two distinct categories: the heart as the pump and the heart that loves.

Webb outlines how the medieval heart is both an organ that propels a person physically through life, and one that can be wounded through emotions and doubt as surely as it can be by arrows or swords. She draws our attention to a thirteenth-century poem by Guido Cavalcanti, which to modern readers may at first appear to be simply an overwrought metaphor about a lover's protests being as wounding as arrows. But Webb exhorts us to understand that, for the medieval writer, those dangerous feelings of protest or sorrow are indeed passing through his body into his alert and thus wounded heart.

Webb effectively argues that medieval thinkers believed the heart was the body's true sovereign, its ruler, and not the brain as understood by modern scientists. The heart was thought to have a respiratory function, but medieval people pictured it as a flow of airborne spirits to the heart, making the heart the seminal heat generator for the body. For all the thinkers of the Middle Ages, the heart is the seat of the soul.

We see the heart played a minor role in medical treatment in the Middle Ages, but it was most important to philosophers, poets, and clerics. Medieval thinkers could not separate the physical and the metaphysical aspects of the heart, and so, for them, the sign—the physical need for the heart—and the symbol—its emotional resonance—were inextricably intertwined. We can see this from the telling story of Saint Clare of Montefalco.

In August 1308 at the monastery of Santa Croce in Montefalco, Italy, the abbess Chiara Vengente dies. Throughout her life she had many visions, and she insisted Christ had visited her, and dwelt in her heart. Though the temperature and humidity were high when she died, her body resisted decay. At her death, the sisters took her heart out of the body and put it in a box. A few days later they opened the box and then opened her heart. They found a tiny sculptural image of Christ on the Cross not wrought from the precious metals of gold or silver but from the very flesh of the heart. This relic has been venerated for centuries, and is still on display at the Basilica of Saint Clare in Montefalco.

This story encapsulates much of the thinking about the heart in the Middle Ages. Webb's study and its excellent bibliography document the philosophical, theological, political, and poetic medieval texts devoted to cardiac function at all levels of understanding. Despite their fascination with the heart as an object, medieval thinkers' veneration of the heart is more about God than the body, and more about philosophy and theology than about biology and physiology.

Though modern students might scoff at the limited understanding of the medieval scholars of the heart and its place in their cosmological order, they still have lessons for us as we try to get our hands around the continuing importance of the symbolic heart.

The two-lobed heart symbol that we know today became ubiquitous in the medieval period, and that shape, as representative of all the heart may mean, has persevered. For people of the Middle Ages, the heart is the very center of all aspects of their world—their religious faiths, their families, their lovers, their kings. Even today in my cardiology practice, I listen to my patients to understand how they center their hearts. How patients relate to their own lives—companions they bring to appointments, or stories they tell about their work, hobbies, or faith—will inevitably be an integral component of how they relate to their physical heart and its state of disease or health. We have much more scientific information about the heart's biology and physical importance, but the centrality of the heart to our emotional lives is not as far from the ideas of the medieval scholars as we might like to imagine.

Just after the medieval period, a European scholar made a surprising assertion that should have radically changed Western Europeans' cardiovascular understanding. Michael Servetus, a Renaissance humanist who lived from 1511 to 1553 CE, is given credit, in our era, for the description of the pulmonary circulation. Servetus was a polymath versed in many sciences including mathematics, astronomy, human anatomy, medicine, and multiple languages. His book *Christianismi Restitutio* contained a section on physiology which outlined his analysis of the circulation of blood through the lungs. The book also contained his refutations of the French reformer John Calvin's theology and that of the Catholic Church's strict doctrine regarding the Holy Trinity and the nature of Christ's divinity. Because of those heresies—to both Catholic and newly formed Protestant institutions—the book was banned and all known copies burned. For all his genius and skills, Servetus was burned at the stake during the Protestant Reformation in Switzerland where he had fled from France to hide from the Catholic Church's persecution.

A century later William Harvey, in 1628, was left to complete the circle, publishing the treatise that became the pulmonary and circulatory breakthrough of Western Europe.

E' trasse poi de li occhi tuo' sospiri,
  i qua' me saettò nel cor sì forte,
  ch'i' mi partì sbigotito fuggendo.

Love pulled sighs from your eyes,
shooting them into my heart so strongly
that I fled, confounded.

—Guido Cavalcanti

ISLAMIC MEDICINE

The Eastern Roman Empire, Byzantium, lasted for one thousand years, with its most powerful years extending from 476 to 732 CE. This Roman Empire in the East lasted considerably longer than that in the West. While the Eastern Empire was immensely wealthy, it eventually degenerated into luxury and sloth. Nevertheless, a series of brilliant physicians helped save the Greek and Alexandrian medical writings even as the capital, Constantinople, was starved of economic and intellectual resources as the empire gradually collapsed.

The slow fall of the Eastern Roman Empire is counterbalanced by the flourishing of the Islamic period, which begins in 732 CE and continues through various dynasties and empires through 1500 CE, generally considered the end of the medieval Islamic period. The lands controlled by various caliphates during this time covered the Ancient Near East and much of the southern Mediterranean coast, extending into the Iberian Peninsula to the west and through the Arabian Peninsula to the east.

These centuries saw, throughout this area, a procession of brilliant Arabic, Persian, Syrian, and Jewish physicians, prominently Rhazes, Albucasis, Avicenna, and Moses Maimonides. In the broadest sense all these thinkers taught that the heart was central to any understanding of the body. The heart was considered the prince of the body and the seat of the soul, while the lungs fanned the heart, and the liver was the guardian of the heart, adjacent to the stomach and the gallbladder, which together were considered the seat of pleasure.

As we can see, this thinking is in keeping with Aristotle's assertions about the heart's importance. This approach treats the heart as the physical, emotional, and political center of the body. Their physiological understanding is, like Western Europe's at this time, rooted in Aristotle's concepts of the four humors, and it preserves the concept as the four basic conditions of the heart: hot, cold, dry, and wet.

The medical giant of this period is Avicenna, a Persian by birth. Born in 980 CE, he was a child prodigy who by the age of ten had memorized the Quran and all the books then taught in the schools. Over the next six years he studied jurisprudence, philosophy, natural sciences, logic, and Euclidian geometry. At age eighteen, he was so famous as a physician that he was called upon to treat the ruler of Persia.

Avicenna's concept of heart disease is metaphysical and not scientific. Like his predecessors, he embraced the humoral concepts of the Greek medicine. At this time, Arabic medicine's entire physiological process was governed and directed by a conceptual division of the body's processes into three basic faculties: the natural faculty, which is the soul; the animal faculty, which is the vital source of life; and the mental faculty, which embodies cognition.

Regarding the heart, we need only concern ourselves with the animal mandate that ensures life, and is manifest in systole, or compression, and diastole, or relaxation, of the heart muscle. For Avicenna, the vital animal faculty is located in the heart and this faculty then reaches the organs by way of the arteries to give them life.

The heart and the animal power produce anger and loftiness, though other, less visceral emotions are considered to be part of the mental faculty. Anger is the surging of the heart's blood and the emergence of innate heat on the body surface.

The psychic and psychological ailments of the heart and Avicenna's suggested remedies were a new contribution to medicine. These were built around the cardiac spirit (i.e., animal spirit or power) and its many manifestations.

In short, Avicenna bases all physical states upon the qualities of the spirit, themselves dependent upon spirit-generating elements—such as blood, phlegm, bile, and black bile—and on temperamental states of heat, cold, moisture, and dryness, corresponding to Aristotle's humors.

The medieval Islamic world's understanding of the circulation of the blood deserves distinct consideration. Arabic medicine had continued to accept Galen's erroneous belief in microscopic pores in the interventricular septum allowing the blood to pass between the left and right ventricles.

The greatest contribution to the circulation of the heart and lungs belongs to Ibn al-Nafis, who lived from 1213 to 1288 CE, in the regions around Syria and Egypt. Refuting Galen's porous septum concept, Ibn al-Nafis accurately described the pulmonary circulation centuries before Servetus and Harvey in Europe. Aristotle's and Galen's writings, however, held remarkable sway. Their ideas remained widespread and, though less accurate than Ibn al-Nafis's, held out as the dominant approach, though some researchers have recently suggested that Ibn al-Nafis's theories about the pulmonary system may have made their way through scholars and across empires to have reached Michael Servetus as a young student, inspiring his writings on those same systems.

Other diseases of the heart observed and described during this period include cardiac abscess, pericardial effusion, differentiation of chest pain similar to stomach pain from severe chest pain leading to death, arrhythmias occurring in the young and the elderly as well as in healthy individuals, and pericarditis.

Out of these observations a complex system of diagnosis and treatment of the heart evolves and is used with a host of treatments both pharmaceutical and nonpharmaceutical throughout the Islamic world.

Medieval Islamic medicine formed the roots from which modern Western medicine arose. At the same time, much like their Western counterparts and precursors, Islamic practitioners recognized the symbolic importance of the heart before grasping the physiology of its functions. Throughout human history, the metaphorical understanding comes first, and we cannot escape the import of how our ancestors, near and far, have navigated that primordial symbolic understanding of the heart.

ANCIENT INDIAN MEDICINE

To understand the ancient medical knowledge of the subcontinent of India we must begin when Indo-European tribes—an Eastern branch of Indo-Iranians, or Aryans, already established in ancient Iran—migrated through the passes of Afghanistan into the Indus Valley in the second millennium BCE. This area is a small northwestern part of India, a huge continent over one and one half million square miles. In antiquity, when man had a more personal relationship with nature, the Indus River Valley was an ideal place to settle. A vibrant civilization predating the Aryans was found by archaeologists in 1920. This city of Mohenjo Daro, built on the banks of the Indus River, has left literary records that can no longer be read. We are left with archaeology finds dated to 3000–2500 BCE which tell us that the Indus River civilization was contemporary with Egypt and Mesopotamia.

Of course we should like to know what kind of medicine the Indus people practiced, but, alas, there have as yet been found no texts or pertinent documents; their medicine would most likely have been similar to other peoples' in the third millennium BCE—that is, a combination of religion, magic, and empirical treatment.

Archaeological findings reveal the advanced public health and sanitation they developed and practiced. Mohenjo Daro had no palaces, temples, or mansions for the rich. The streets were lined with two-story baked-brick houses, which included bathrooms. Rainwater was drained into the street through gutters of pottery and probably also wood. Rubbish was drained by chutes through the wall into tanks for emptying. Because of the lack of translated written evidence, modern scholars do not know whether they understood the use of these sanitation tools as crucial to their personal and collective physical health. Nevertheless, their sanitation practices must have been an important development in their lives.

The Aryans were of Indo-European origin and their language was a Vedic form of Sanskrit, which means it can be read, as it has been passed down and in use since the second century BCE. These languages and a highly developed religion united the people.

What of Vedic medicine?

The primary source used to understand this early people's medical knowledge is the Vedas, their religious and educational texts (the word itself means "knowledge" and "sacred lore"). The texts consist of hymns, prayers, chants, and religious formulas. We can tease out of the Vedas a few medical facts.

According to the Vedas, the gods could cause illness. Rudra is one of many such gods. Rudra's special way of inflicting pain was to shoot arrows into the victim. The arrow, and thus the pain and illness, is removed by prayer, such as: "The arrow that Rudra did cast upon thee, into thy limbs and into thy heart; this here we do draw away from thee."

Varuna, a guardian of law and order, could send all kinds of diseases. Dropsy, in particular, was attributed to him. Dropsy is swelling of the feet and legs, and we know now it is a sign of congestive heart failure. As treatment, the dropsical patient was put in a hut where two rivers came together. A prayer is recited; the patient washes with three branches of grass, and the grass is dipped in water as another prayer is recited.

Vedic medicine could acknowledge these physical signs and symptoms of cardiac function, but at this stage, the practice of cardiology remained entirely within religious ceremonies and practices.

The most complete and in-depth paper on Vedic and post-Vedic medicine is the article "Cardiovascular System and Its Diseases in Ancient Indian Literature" by J. N. Sharma, which translates passages related to the heart and blood vessels. As Sharma notes, the *Rig Veda*, an early religious narrative from 4000 BCE, describes inspiration ("food" being oxygen) and expiration ("waste" being carbon dioxide). The *Atharva Veda*, written three thousand to four thousand years ago, deals with blood vessel anatomy. Through these early texts we can see that there is an attempt to understand the medical importance of how the heart functions, though always through the medium of religion. In the post-Vedic period, from around 1000 BCE, the *Charak Samhita* describes the heart as having cavities (chambers) six hundred years before Hippocrates's similar description.

Charaka, the author of the *Charak Samhita*, observed all functions are dependent on the heart—including the central nervous system. He describes the blood vessels coming off the heart and understood the difference between arteries, which are pulsatile and carry blood away from the heart; veins, which go toward the heart and do not pulse; and capillaries, the tiny vessels that ooze, rather than pulse.

There is no better early description of bacterial endocarditis—bacterial infection of the heart—with embolization of the infected tissue than the one found in the *Charak Samhita*.

The *Charak Samhita* also includes descriptions compatible with cardiac syncope (fainting) and angina pectoris (pressure in the chest from blocked arteries), and the text accurately blames fatty deposits for heart disease, which we now know to be caused by high cholesterol.

To conclude from this history: all archaic medicine is a mixture of magic, religion, and empiric observation. Like the ancient civilizations of Mesopotamia, Egypt, Greece, and Rome, the Indus Valley civilizations described many normal and abnormal cardiac functions, but an enduring reliance on religion and magic remained an obstacle to reliable treatment methods for all peoples from these past millennia.

These are the antecedents of the next phase of Indian medicine, namely Ayurvedic medicine. The roots of Ayurvedic medicine reach back into early Indian medical and religious history as discussed above. In the post-Vedic period Ayurvedic medicine emerges with more anatomic and physiologic observations that will ultimately influence the Greek and Roman way of thinking.

Ayurvedic medicine leans heavily on the teachings of Buddha, who was born circa 400 BCE, and died at age eighty. While the Buddha's teachings are primarily philosophical, the temples that became centers for Buddhist study and worship also became centers of education and research. Central to the maintenance of Ayurvedic tradition was a cadre of well-defined and educated medical professionals. A few of their texts have survived, with the oldest dating from early in the Common Era.

According to the Ayurvedic tradition, the element of wind was the life force which caused movement within the human body. Working through its headquarters (chambers) in the heart (the central organ of the body), "wind" pushed food that had gone into the stomach into the body and through various phases formed fat, muscle, blood, and bone.

The importance of the heart (called *mahat*) was analogous to the king's palace. In addition to being the seat of the human soul (the immutable force, and the male force) mahat also contained the mind, which sent out directions to all other elements of the body. The heart was understood as the body's control center, not the brain as we are taught today.

These records allow us to see that the heart in ancient India, like the heart in ancient Western European and African civilizations, is seen as the most important organ. Early observations attempted to cure cardiac problems such as dropsy, and even as medical observations and understanding increased over time, the heart remained the organ most important to the body in each system of medicine. The poetry that grows out of these cultures reiterates this centrality, treating the heart as the center of emotion and love. As Ayurvedic medicine solidifies the heart as the physical control center of the body, the poetry of Sūrdās shows the heart continues to be seen as the center of self.

His quick and flickering movements captured my mind—
My gaze froze, my mind glazed—
And I quite forgot my body as he studied his reflection;
My heart was cooled with every kind of joy.

~~

The Lord of Sūrdās: Why has he left me now—
Now that he's claimed my heart.

~~

Night comes riding that chariot of the mind, desire,
but morning comes and magnifies pain,
bringing on the fate of Sūrdās's Lord:
day, the thief that steals away
their wealth, these two—the heart

King Kama's land is an intoxicating place—
Strength of mind cannot dwell there,
Nor peace of heart.

What pleasure to my heart.
His innocent childish games!
For all of Gokul he's life breath and wealth;
For his foes, a thorn at the heart.

—Sūrdās
Hindu poet, sixteenth century CE

MESOAMERICA AND THE AMERICA INDIANS

The title of this section is potentially misleading, simply because the Aztecs dominate any discussion of the history of this part of the world. Much of the information that comes down to us begins with Cortés's defeat of the Aztec empire in the early sixteenth century. The spirit of the Catholic priests and Spanish viceroys who followed his conquest to variously shape, destroy, or preserve the history of the Aztec people has greatly determined the extent of the information now available to study and work with.

The Aztecs and the Incas were the well-established, wide-ranging civilizations that greeted the Spanish conquistadors on their arrivals in Central and South America in the sixteenth century. Before these civilizations arose, there were many others, from even before the Mayan and Olmec settlements of Central America and the Nazca settlements on the Peruvian coast, all in the second century BCE. Other civilizations continually arose, through the Toltecs of the tenth, eleventh, and twelfth centuries CE, and beyond.

The definitive historian of the Spanish conquests of these areas, William H. Prescott, provides an overview of the conquistadors' records of the cultures of the Incas and the Aztecs in his two multivolume works from the nineteenth century. His *History of the Conquest of Peru* discusses the plants used by the Inca far to the south, in modern Peru, with no direct reference to use in medicines except for tobacco and cocoa. In his *History of the Conquest of Mexico*, he discusses medicinal plants grown in Montezuma's garden, but provides no direct references to herbals for cardiac use.

Popular culture has given us the easily exaggerated image of Aztec priests, with long, blood-matted hair, standing atop a truncated pyramid as a line of doomed prisoners filed upward to be seized by the head, hand, and foot and placed spread-eagled over a convex sacrificial stone. The prisoner's bare chest is conveniently arched, his ribs expanded, and with a black obsidian knife the still beating heart was extracted by the priest. The heart was held high and placed before the insatiable sun god. While the details of these images may be historically accurate, the complexities of this historic ritual are often reduced to a grossly misleading picture of barbarism. The ritual sacrifice was only one small facet of this very advanced civilization that built pyramids and buildings almost equal to that of ancient Egypt. Furthermore, the Aztec sacrifices—unlike the circuses of death staged in the Roman Colosseum—were not mere spectacles to entertain the populace. These rituals were conducted to keep the sun moving across the heavens as it must, to guarantee the safe continuation of life for the community of believers.

The ancient Aztecs and other Mexican civilizations conceived the sun as the source of all vital force. The name of the sun god worshipped through the sacrifice described above is Ipalnemohuani, a name which means "He by whom all men live." If the god bestowed life on the world, according to his followers, he needed to receive life from it. As the heart is the seat and symbol of life, bleeding hearts of men and animals were presented to the sun god to maintain his strength in order to guide his path across the sky. These sacrifices were magical, not merely religious, and designed not so much to please him but to renew his energy to produce heat, light, and motion.

The Aztec were not the only people to conceive of physical sacrifice and organ consumption as a transfer of power. Similar customs evolved in other parts of the world. In Lagos, West Africa, when a king died his head was cast off and sent to his successor, who ate part of his deceased heart to ensure wisdom and bravery. The Indians of Guayaquil in Ecuador sacrificed men and sowed their fields with the blood and hearts of the sacrificed in hope of a good harvest.

These few examples show the Aztecs were not alone in their cannibalism. There are many more examples of this nature recorded in the literature.

The Aztecs were more than murderous cannibals, though that is how they are often portrayed in modern narratives. Alongside their ritual sacrifices, they developed advanced medical care and their physicians were superior to European doctors at the time of Cortés.

Several important codexes come down to us from the late eighteenth century that describe the drugs used by the Aztecs. There were approximately two thousand different plants in the garden of Montezuma—the last Aztec emperor—in 1519, when the Spanish invaded. From the limited records preserved by the few Spanish monks who chose to preserve texts rather than destroy them as heathen artifacts, it is clear that the Aztecs had established medications and practices to treat many different kinds of recognized illnesses, including many cardiac disorders.

Heart pains had many treatments in Aztec medicine. They could be relieved by the ingestion of the ash of a stag's burned heart and a medicine brewed from both the flower and the bark of the Mexican magnolia (*Talauma mexicana*) called *yoloxóchitl*, or heart flower, in the Nahuatl language. Alternatively, a plant called *nonochton* was used. The plant is found growing near ants' nests. Ground up with a burned heart of a deer once again, but also with the metal gold and the alloy electrum, as well as three other items—two stones called *teoxihuitl* and *chichiltic tapachtli*, and another plant called *tetlahuitl*—they can be mixed with water and drunk as a cure.

Through their various cures, we can see they distinguished between different kinds of chest pain—they had separate treatments for chest tightness and for a burning sensation in the chest, which may be what we call heartburn today. For this heartburn, there was a recipe for taking the juice of a root called *tlaca-camotli*, mixing it with ground pearls, crystals, and other stones, and drinking this mixture. A treatment specifically for chest tightness uses a plant called *tlat lacotic*, instructing patients to wash the plant's root in hot water, macerate it, and then drink the juice as an emetic, to induce vomiting.

The Aztecs' medications combined many different approaches, including empirically medicinal herbs and even magical ingestion of representative stones and organs. The importance of the heart appears through their physicians' trial-and-error recognition of cardiac diseases, as well as the symbolic importance of the use of a strong heart from a strong animal, such as a stag, to treat the ailing human heart in need of an inflow of strength.

It may be difficult to believe but until the sixteenth century no one had been known to draw, paint, or sculpt an anatomically accurate image of the human heart—not the Egyptians, Chinese, Greeks, Roman, Arabs, or Ottomans—until Andreas Vesalius in 1543 published his study of anatomy with an accurate picture of the heart (crucially without Galen's porous interventricular septum).

However, there exists an Olmec clay effigy of a human figure holding an enlarged anatomically correct heart. This Olmec potter lived 2,500 years before Vesalius. The Olmecs thrived from around 1400 to 400 BCE, in the hills of what is now Las Bocas in Pueblo, southeast of Mexico City. The Olmec, like the Aztec, knew what the heart looked like because they opened the chest to extract the heart, probably to appease their sun god.

For Mesoamerican people, as for so many other early cultures, the heart is a symbol of strength and life. Ingesting it imbues the priest—and therefore the god—with strength, and thus the sun would keep coming up. For the Aztecs, the heart connects people with the whole of life, beyond the life of the singular self.

We must not forget Aztec civilization was so much more than ritual slaughter and cannibalism. Herbals and medicine were quite advanced. While they were sacrificing people as part of religious rituals, they were still respecting the need for the heart to function properly. They knew some herbs caused the heart to be quieter, some stronger, and some relieved cardiac pain.

The visionary vocabulary of their language produced poetry, and the remaining records include at least one poem incorporating the heart. Through both religious ritual and poetry the Aztec recounted what was dear to them. All poems and songs dedicated to the gods were very consequential for them. The patron god of poets was Xochipilli. As many poems reveal, the heart could be happy, strong, colorful, or even made of stone.

The Mayan language, as well, has many metaphors of the heart. These linguistic phrases were preserved by an unknown Dominican friar who traveled to the New World from Spain, arriving in the state of Chiapas, Mexico, around 1592. He compiled a dictionary to aid his fellow priests in converting the pagan Indians to Christianity. He tracked down native terms for over ten thousand Spanish words. In the Tzotzil languages he found "infinite expressions" derived from the word *heart*. To list a few:

> my heart cries
> my heart grows small
> my heart hurts
> my heart withdraws
> my heart becomes two
> my heart aches
> my heart is clamoring

American Indian medical practices before the Europeans arrived have often been overlooked or ignored, and often consigned to obscurity. A brief summary can provide a window into their medical practices and their view of the heart.

What we do know is that ancient American Indians' mythology and spiritual life was rich and endowed with symbolism. Their medicine followed their religion—a nature worship filled with mysticism and ceremony. Yet mixed with mysticism and magic was a profound knowledge of animals and plant life.

The Indians knew very little about the circulatory system but knew the heart caused the flow of blood, and some tribes distinguished between arteries and veins. The story of Sky Woman, as it comes to us from the Anishinaabe and the Haudenosaunee, is an excellent representation of American Indians' understanding of the physical and symbolic roles of the heart and of the importance of its physical health.

In the story, a pregnant Sky Woman jumps into a hole and falls to the human world from hers, far above. As she falls, she reaches out to trees and plants she passes, gathering seeds that will ultimately help the people in the human world. Sky Woman eventually lands safely, thanks to the birds and animals who assist her. Eventually she gives birth to her daughter, who grows up and herself gives birth to twins. Sadly, Sky Woman's daughter dies in the difficult childbirth, but when her body is buried, important medicinal plants grow up from her body, which has itself become their seeds. Among these medicinal gifts are strawberries, which grow from her heart.

It may at first appear that strawberries are linked to the heart for many early American Indians because of their physical resemblance to the organ. But strawberries, their fruit and more importantly their edible leaves and stems, are an accurate traditional pharmaceutical treatment for diabetes and heart disease.

Along with the Anishinaabe's use of strawberries, there are four examples of herbals consciously used for cardiac stimulus by other groups in North America. The North Carolina Indian groups used holly, *Ilex vomitoria*. The Winnebago and the Dakota tribes to their north used horsemint, also known as spotted bee balm, *Monarda punctata*. The Delaware used pokeweed, or Virginia poke, *Phytolacca americana*, while the Pawnee preferred to use bush morning glory, *Ipomoea leptophylla*, as a cardiac treatment.

Peripheral edema, or dropsy, due to congestive heart failure was not uncommon in American Indians, and they effectively used diuretics they cultivated in their areas. For the Plains tribes, sumac, *Rhus copallinum*, was the preferred treatment, while the Winnebago and the Dakota used spotted wintergreen, *Chimaphila maculata*. The Ottawa and the Chippewa used *Xanthorhiza simplicissima*, shrub yellowroot. The Plains tribes used sarsaparilla and bigleaf magnolia, while the Tewa, in the Pueblo area, used the juniper *Juniperus monosperma*.

Like the civilizations of the classical western world, the early peoples throughout the Americas understood the importance of the heart on many levels. They sought ways to treat cardiac pain and ways to improve cardiac function, and they constructed narratives and rituals to acknowledge the centrality of the heart's importance to emotional strength and well-being, not just in the individual, but in the greater world that the community itself inhabits. The heart keeps us alive, and the heart keeps the sun moving across the sky.

The mature man:
a heart as firm as stone
a wise countenance
the owner of a face and a heart
who is capable of understanding.
            —*Huehuetlatolli*, The Orations of the Elders

EASTERN ASIAN MEDICINE

At the end of the Cultural Revolution, in 1986, I had the rare opportunity to give a series of lectures on cardiology at Fujian Medical College and Hospital. I learned and absorbed more than I was able to give in return. Chinese medicine is complex, and for me to try and integrate all their historic areas of study, including acupuncture with its maze of meridians, complex pulse lore, or their incredible knowledge of herbal medicine, would require several lifetimes of study.

The oldest recorded records in China can be traced to the Shang dynasty existing along the Huang He, or the Yellow River, in the northeast section of Henan Province, flourishing especially during the eighteenth through sixteenth centuries BCE. The Shang dynasty left traces of medical treatment, but no definitive records of diagnosis or medicines.

In the West we are most familiar with the traditional concept of the yin and the yang. This concept describing the necessary balance of life forces is a key component of both Chinese philosophy and traditional Chinese medicine. The concept of this dualism began as a tool of divination, reaching recorded prominence in the fourth century BCE and was further developed as a philosophical approach during the period of Confucianism (Confucius, c. 551 to c. 478 BCE). Its vitality and importance as a philosophy and as the basis of traditional medicinal approaches such as acupuncture continue to the present day.

In this worldview, life is comprised of two forces, yin and yang, that are constitutionally opposite but must always work in tandem with each other. In traditional medicine, as in numerous philosophical approaches that arose throughout the history of East Asia, the path to health and harmony is found in balancing these forces in the body and the mind.

In addition to the concepts of yin and yang, traditional Chinese medicine also ascribes five phases to the world at large. These phases, like the four Greek elements and their respective humors, base the description of anatomical functions in an elemental description of the world itself. The elements and their corresponding organs are linked together in the search for balance, and thus health: wind is associated with the lungs, humidity with the spleen, wood with the liver, and water with the kidney. The heart is represented by fire.

In the case of the heart, the physician who understood the body through the five phases might realize the patient was harmed by heat confined to the heart. The physician would say the heart was being hit by evil. However, if the heart's heat or pain continued, and thus was subject to a secondary infection, the physician would have to determine the source of the evil influence. Like the other ancient cultures, the ancient Chinese navigated the physical symptoms they observed through overwhelmingly magical understandings of their evil influences.

Examination of the patient's body was not as obviously available as it may sound to us. Though empirical observations were crucial for early practitioners, at that time it was indecent to touch the body of a person of a different sex; the only part of the body that could be felt was the pulse taken at the wrist.

Pulse diagnosis dates back to the fourth century BCE. Over the centuries Chinese physicians became masters of pulse diagnosis. The systems developed were intricate and convoluted and took years to learn and master. Despite the rigorous analysis they applied to the pulse, its variations, and its symptoms, the practitioners did not ultimately connect the pulse to the heart. Chinese pulse lore was inordinately complex and all-encompassing.

An important component of Chinese medicine is the understanding that there exists within the human body a system of channels through which the vital energy and blood are delivered. This system of energy tide is the foundation of the long-standing science of acupuncture but will not be relevant to this study of the heart.

Throughout the centuries the focus on pulse, channels, and balance of yin and yang ultimately meant the anatomic and beating heart was not directly studied. The East and the West arrived at different conclusions.

In the East, health was assessed according to energy channels, while in the West the working of arterial channels was increasingly central to medical practices.

Despite the otherwise overarching focus on the pulse in and of itself, Chinese medical history does include early insight into the arterial system that so fascinated Galen. In the *Huangdi Neijing*, the emperor Huangdi— said to have lived in 2600 BCE, forty centuries before Harvey— wrote: "All the blood is under control of the heart and the blood current flows continuously in a circle and never stops." This early, accurate description was never embraced as a central component of medicine in ancient China.

Though the pulse is a product of the heart's physical function in the body, practitioners did not explore the anatomical connection due to restrictions on both intimate examination and human dissection. Nevertheless, the metaphorical heart was often treated as the center of emotion and thought, as throughout the cultures and histories we have already examined. As early as the third century CE, the poet Xie Lingyun uses the heart as a barometer for feeling and truth, referring to it in parallel with the concept of mind. In the later Buddhist poetry of Hanshan, from the eighth century, we can see the heart is used as a metaphor for the self. In the poetry of Bai Juyi from the same era, the heart is also referred to as a source of emotion. While the pulse and the flow of energy prevails in the history of Chinese medicine, the symbolic heart once again stakes its claim as the most important organ for experiencing life.

The history of Japanese medicine is immensely influenced by the Chinese approach to medicine. To know ancient Japanese medicine is to know Chinese medicine—at least until recent times. Contemporary Japanese cardiovascular research is an important component of world cardiology.

Japanese medicine, throughout its history, has been influenced by other societies' understandings and practices over the centuries, while still preserving its own culture. The periods as they are usually broken down by historians provide an overview of how medicine evolved.

From antiquity to 96 BCE, disease was thought to be caused by, or sent from, the gods. Magical incantations and exorcisms were the primary treatment for illnesses, though the archaeological record also reveals that botanicals—plants, herbs, and flowers—were mixed with rice wine as possible early pharmaceutical treatments.

An important development arises near the end of the First Nara Period of 97 BCE–709 CE. In the fifth century, Japanese rulers establish ties with Korean courts, importing Korean medicinal practices that were heavily influenced by and in many ways derived from Chinese medicinal practices. By the end of the period, Japanese scholars had been sent to China to study medicine, and Buddhism became increasingly prevalent in Japan. A medical school founded on Buddhist principles was opened, and the studies of acupuncture, massage, and moxibustion—a treatment that involves burning herbs on specified parts of the body—were all introduced at this time. Throughout the Second Nara Period, 710–784 CE, Buddhism continued to be a guiding principle in Japanese medical thought.

Throughout the Heian Period, 785–1186 CE, Japanese medical practice closely followed Chinese practice, taking its cues from the established Chinese understandings of energy and balance. Vessels become a part of the conception of human anatomy, with the existence of two sets of vessels—one with blood and one with air, or pneuma—becoming an established belief.

This reliance on China for medical leadership begins to wane during the Kamakura Period, 1187–1333 CE, when a feudalist, military government is established, bringing with it a strong sense of nationalism and a focus on local advances and accomplishments. In the Muromachi Period, 1334–1568 CE, however, the royal hierarchies became increasingly localized, leading to many civil wars fought over land and power. At the end of this period, Portuguese missionaries arrived, and the Jesuit priests introduced and taught Western medical knowledge and practice.

In the wake of these civil wars, the moves toward unity in the Azuchi-Momoyama Period, from 1569 to 1615 CE, saw many changes in medicine. New Japanese medical texts were written, but Chinese texts were still used. Christianity, however, was banned, and European missionaries as well as Portuguese doctors left the country.

The Edo, or Tokugawa, Period, from 1616 to 1867 CE, brought more stability. Doctors at this time relied often on the Sung Period Chinese texts, but more Western-style anatomical investigation was beginning to be explored, as commerce with the Portuguese, Dutch, Spanish, English, and Germans was reestablished, though on limited terms.

From the Meiji Period of 1868 CE through to the present day, Japanese medicine has embraced the modernism brought with industrialization, and Japan is now a world leader in medical treatment and research.

Where and how is the heart represented in all these periods?

Energy, when cited in the classics, is commonly translated as *blood*. The concept of the circulation of blood was known but poorly developed. Energy and blood were considered to circulate together, but had no relation to the heart as the pulsatile organ.

Palpitation, the act of pulse-taking, was highly developed and again relied on Chinese knowledge. The radial artery was used, and through palpitation one could determine not only the condition of the heart and aorta but the state of both storage organs, such as skeletal muscles, and hollow organs, such as the intestines and stomach. Though the pulse could reveal information about the heart, it was revealed as part of the greater physical system as a whole, and was not apparently understood as a direct action of specific cardiac and pulmonary system connections. At the time, examination of the pulse combined with red skin color was associated with a diagnosis of heart disease. An abnormality of the tongue was also used as an aid in diagnosis.

The use of a complete analysis of the pulse's physical attributes, as well as the influence of other physical symptoms, for diagnosis in traditional East Asian medicine is impressive, often revealing otherwise hidden connections between systems. The analysis of the anatomical heart was not, however, a priority, and the heart was not seen explicitly as a pump.

Modern students might assume the emotional or metaphysical role of the heart is less, because the heart is not associated physically as a central component of the body. There are examples in classical Japanese poetry, however, which treat the heart as the seat of emotion, much as in Chinese poetry. In ancient Japanese poetry the metaphor of a broken heart represents sadness and despair—in many ways the same image modern Western poetry employs to this day.

Even when starting from radically different approaches to physical cardiac treatment, human cultures continually return to the heart as a symbol for strong emotion, as well as for connections to community and to life itself.

Once the mind stops striving the world loses importance
Once the heart is content it does not swerve from the truth
                                    — Xie Lingyun
                              (b. 385 CE, China)

My heart's not the same as yours
If your heart was like mine
You'd get it and be right here

                                    —Hanshan
                              (b. 8th cen. CE, China)

My heart's as tangled
as the wild fern patterns

                                    —Minamoto no Tōru
                              (b. 822 CE, Japan)

As the human heart's so fickle
your feelings may have changed

                                    —Ki no Tsurayuki
                              (b.872 CE, Japan)

I had hoped to keep secret
feelings that had begun to stir
within my heart.

                                    —Mibu no Tadami
                              (9th cen. CE, Japan)

"I feel so sorry for you."
No one comes to mind
Who would say that to me,
So I will surely die alone
of a broken heart.

                                    —Fujiwara no Koremasa
                              (b. 924 CE, Japan)

Though my heart shatters
My love rages yet.

—Minamoto no Shigeyuki
(d. 1000 CE, Japan)

There is no escape in this sad world
With a melancholy heart
I enter deep in the mountains

—Fujiwara no Shunzei
(b. 1114 CE, Japan)

FINALE

Bacchus opens the gates of the heart.

—Horace

Humanity has been persistent in looking for the source of a person's emotion and personality. This search is the source of human development in the arts, religion, science, and medicine. Evidence from prehistoric and early historical periods bestows insight into the process of becoming human. Humanity returns again and again to the heart as this possible source. Since history repeats itself, we must study the past to understand the present and make better choices.

Archaeology has followed this path. The early cave paintings—the oldest drawings made by long gone people to survive, uncovered by archaeologists—establish the heart in the framework of even preliterate communities. The heart in the center of the elephant's body aligns the importance of the heart as a physical element, in that it is anatomically powering the animal that presumably must be killed. It also honors its importance as a metaphysical element, in that it is included in the vivid outline that a human, otherwise concerned with safety and survival, took the time to render on the rocky cave wall.

Archaeologists have been amazingly successful in unearthing the act of developing a particular form, as either two- or three-dimensional objects intentionally created by *Homo sapiens* and other ancestors. The Paleolithic cave paintings in southern France and other parts of Western Europe, dating from 10,000 to 34,000 years ago, are two-dimensional. The knapping of stone to make tools, three-dimensional objects, can be traced back 2.6 million years.

The imaginative domain of creating forms is an auspicious way to start. The heart symbol inhabits both two- and three-dimensional forms. Rendered most often in flat, stylized, two-dimensional form, the two-lobed symbol carries with it a three-dimensional complexity and meaning for the observers. Evidence for symbolic behavior extends much further into the past than the records of humanity's emblematic approaches. The meaning of the symbolic heart is difficult to analyze, much less to understand, but I believe we must in order to better understand humanity.

Each culture from our recorded history, whether from Europe or Africa or the Americas or Asia, has established an understanding of the heart as an important, if not the most important, component of a person's physical and emotional being. Ancient people continually recognize the heart's significance before its anatomical function is defined on any level. The metaphysical understanding of the heart—symbolic, emotional—always comes first.

Much as the widow, whose story started me on this journey, thought of her husband's heart primarily in its symbolic role, all human history thinks first of the heart as the center of emotion and thought, and thus of self. Would a widow consider her husband's heart to be the seat of his soul? If so, surely she could not bring herself to bury him without the physical sign that symbolized that crucial part of his very self.

Would many physicians be surprised at this often-overlooked fundamental human conception of the heart? Many cultures and their assumptions underlie all our discourse, conscious or not.

Even a rigorous scientific study about the development of computers as potentially independent thinkers relies on this original belief in the metaphysical function of the heart. Richard Yonck's 2020 work, *Heart of the Machine: Our Future in a World of Artificial Emotional Intelligence*, associates the heart with emotions in the title itself. Nowhere in his book is the heart discussed as a functioning pump, nor is the word explicitly mentioned in its metaphysical sense. There is a detailed discussion of the physical brain, exploring the intricacies of emotional connections and hormonal responses. Yet the title of his book crushes the totality of his thesis. The first word in the title, the word chosen to signal all the complex import of the ways that computers must work to capture humanity, is *heart*. This intelligent scientist falls into the trap of using a word codified in all the ancient societies examined here. So often, scientists have the audacity to use the word *heart* in all its symbolic meaning, employing the implicit metaphysical connections with which all of human history has imbued our symbol. Even for these rationalists, the heart represents love, faith, humility, hope, kindness, beauty, gentleness, compassion, and strength— just to mention a few of the many attributes we have seen throughout our many-faceted cultural histories. When science asks patients or readers to discount all of the hidden meaning when it comes to the physical heart, we must acknowledge that such a shift is a much greater leap than we are admitting, for our patients and for the physicians themselves.

As a practicing physician, I understand that even the earliest moments of my life can influence how I interpret my patient's history. Even at times more directly than I expected. A recent patient recognized me from my days as a camp counselor and athletic field director, and he greeted me as Captain Moose, just as he had when he was a camper. As the basketball counselor, I'd urged the camp owner to install a shorter-than-regulation backboard to the side of the basketball court to allow the youngest campers the enjoyment of a successful shot. As I took my patient's history, he told me this story. During the camp season, there was a big field day where all the campers competed in a relay of activities. His role had been to make five free throws at that shorter goal so the team could move to their next event. He still remembered sinking them in only six tries, and how his teammates cheered. He told me that day was a turning point in his life. Listening to his story, I understood that his physical concerns were not just about the function of his heart as a pump, but also that they were bound up in his view of himself and his history of activity and accomplishment.

Like my patient, I look back on my time at that summer camp as some of the most important years of my life. The friendships I made have lasted for decades, and the leadership roles that counselors and campers were encouraged to take on opened new experiences to us all. I thought, all those years ago, that my time at camp taught me to work with kids, but really, it taught me to work with people: to set heights a person needs to reach, and to help a person find their path for success. Contemporary cardiologists have made herculean leaps in understanding the complex nature of the heart and its function in the body, but humanity's approach to what the heart means to us emotionally has scarcely changed over centuries. Our approach to life and death, illness and recovery, is still filtered through all our historical associations. While an electrocardiogram measures the electrical activity of the heart, a youthful memory of a summer camp success, when closely listened to, helps me understand the nuanced changes and fears that a patient brings to my office.

Do I have a valid thesis? The heart has both physical and metaphysical importance—the accurate medical attention to each is key to any physician who treats the physical heart.

Is the heart truly the one *Homo sapiens* organ capable of sustaining our species?

Over the past two billion years millions of species have perished, but I have never read where any species disappeared by their own action. Predators, starvation, and natural disasters ended their sojourn on planet Earth, but not their own wishes or their own actions. Human emotions, however, have often led us to make destructive decisions—we are in the midst of a climate crisis brought about by our own inabilities to limit dangerous production and consumption on a societal level, and we allow our governments to stockpile and prepare to deploy ostensibly defensive weapons that would destroy our habitat on a planetary scale. *Homo sapiens* has the ability to destroy itself with nuclear weapons and other physical means. This skill comes from the brain, not the heart. And yet we symbolically grant the heart the power over the emotions that urge us to defend ourselves, or to see others as an enemy, or even to make peace with our neighbors on any scale.

To answer my question: Do I have a valid scientific thesis? Modern medicine would tell us no, because this is not a double-blind placebo-controlled trial. This style of evaluating treatment results based entirely on measured outcomes has its place, and is often useful. But too often the primacy of double-blind control results obscures other types of useful results. Many preeminent observers in history did not have the benefit of two distinct populations to compare and contrast when they made their scientific leaps of understanding. Archaeology has fallen under the spell of prioritizing results that are able to be measured the most precisely. In the excitement of being able to accurately chart and measure and carbon-date each shard and shell and rock and layer of a four-foot-square area of a dig, the detail gets so small that the big picture gets lost.

In our rush to measure the physical heart and all its functions, we must not overlook the symbolic heart and its accompanying concerns. In our rush to provide the most up-to-date statistics for a chance of longer life, we must also acknowledge a patient's metaphysical concerns. A study can tell us that a medication can improve the chance of a healthy outcome by a small percent, but can it tell us about how the patient will navigate the next years of life? All the anxiety and money potentially spent for very little effect, and without looking at the big picture. We must be wary of relying so heavily on the physical measurements that we forget our patients' metaphysical hearts.

A researcher can't get a paper published without a control.

Of course, there is no possible double-blind trial that could measure the strength or the importance of the symbolic heart.

So, in lieu of such a trial, I accumulated the stories of many societies—some quite ancient, most seen as medically primitive by our twenty-first-century standards.

But what I have concluded: Their myths, legends, tales, poetry all originate in the heart. Whether the heart is understood as an organ that moves blood or not, the heart remains continually the repository of our humanity.

The widow of the patient gave the doctors clear instructions. Find her husband's heart, put it back in his chest, then bury him. They did as she asked. And her metaphysical heartache was eased and she was satisfied and at peace.

The author of this tome is a physician trained to treat mechanical afflictions of the heart. But I must remember that all of my patients know intuitively the symbolic heart—so to effectively treat my patient, the emotional, philosophical, and psychological components of the illness must be openly addressed.

To close this endeavor let us harken back to earlier in this essay to the importance of the collective consciousness revealed by Freud, Jung, and their disciples. They so brilliantly refocused our attention to the beauty of the metaphysical heart. The heart has become the center of our emotions through evolution. Human knowledge and emotional fulfillment are encoded into our genes.

I hope my study of these many cultures and the history of the symbolic heart has helped me relieve the anxiety every patient experiences when asked to see a "cardiologist."

REFERENCES AND FURTHER READING

If this account of the symbolic heart has given you any pleasure, please think kindly of the man who wrote it. On the other hand, if I only succeeded in boring you, please believe I did not do it on purpose.

For each section I provide the references I relied on for my thoughts.

Also enclosed is a longer list of my favorite studies and useful references for surveying the heart as it was understood before William Harvey. There are, of course, a multitude of individual journal articles and many volumes about this subject. I hope the sources listed here can provide you with a place to start.

Introduction

Ashdown, Raymond R., and Stanley H. Done. *Color Atlas of Veterinary Anatomy: The Ruminants*. Vol. 1. Baltimore: University Park Press, 1984.

Harvey, William. *The Anatomical Exercises on the Motion of the Heart and Blood in Animals*. Frankfort, 1628.

Hawkes, Jacquetta, ed. *The World of the Past*. New York: Alfred A. Knopf, 1963.

Jayasinghe, Seroj. "Complexity Science to Conceptualize Health and Disease: Is it Relevant to Clinical Medicine?" *Mayo Clinic Proceedings* 87, no. 4 (April 2012): 314–319.

Stolberg, Sheryl Gay. "On Medicine's Frontier: The Last Journey of James Quinn." *New York Times*, October 8, 2002, Science.

White, Paul Dudley, and Helen Donovan. *Hearts: Their Long Follow-Up*. Philadelphia: W. B. Saunders, 1967.

The Symbolic Heart

Boyadjian, N. *The Heart: Its Symbolism, Its Iconography, and Its Diseases*. Antwerp: Esco, 1985.

Breuil, Abbé H. *Quatre cents siècles d'art pariétal; les cavernes ornées de l'âge du renne*. Montignac, Dordogne: Centre d'Études et de Documentation Préhistoriques, 1952.

Clottes, Jean. *Chauvet Cave: The Art of Earliest Times*. Translated by Paul G. Bahn. Salt Lake City: University of Utah Press, 2003.

Darwin, Charles. *The Expression of the Emotions in Man and Animals.* London, 1872.

Fordham, Frieda. *An Introduction to Jung's Psychology.* New York: Penguin, 1966.

Hillman, James. *A Blue Fire: Selected Writings.* Edited by Thomas Moore. New York: Harper, 1989.

———. *The Thought of the Heart and the Soul of the World.* Woodstock, CT: Spring, 1996.

Jung, Carl G., ed. *Man and His Symbols.* New York: Dell, 1968.

Jung, Carl. G. *The Undiscovered Self: The Dilemma of the Individual in Society.* Translated by R. F. C. Hall. New York: New American Library, 2006.

Lewis-Williams, David. *The Mind in the Cave: Consciousness and the Origins of Art.* London: Thames & Hudson, 2002.

Renfrew, Colin, and Iain Morley, eds. *Image and Imagination: A Global Prehistory of Figurative Representation.* Cambridge, UK: McDonald Institute for Archaeological Research, 2007.

Ronnberg, Ami, and Kathleen Martin, eds. *The Book of Symbols: Reflections on Archetypal Images.* Köln: Taschen, 2010.

Sells, Benjamin, ed. *Working with Images: The Theoretical Base of Archetypal Psychology.* Woodstock, CT: Spring, 2000.

Snyder, Peter J., Rebecca Kaufman, John Harrison, and Paul Maruff. "Charles Darwin's Emotional Expression 'Experiment' and His Contribution to Modern Neuropharmacology." *Journal of the History of the Neurosciences* 19, no. 2 (April 2010): 158–170.

The Heart in Religion

Acierno, Louis J. *The History of Cardiology*. London: Parthenon, 1994.

Al-Janziyya, Ibn Qayyim. *Medicine of the Prophet*. Translated by Penelope Johnstone. Cambridge: Islamic Texts Society, 1998.

Bellah, Robert N. *Religion in Human Evolution: From the Paleolithic to the Axial Age*. Cambridge, MA: Harvard University Press, 2011.

Brim, Charles J. *Medicine in the Bible: The Pentateuch Torah*. New York: Froben, 1936.

Gordon, Benjamin Lee. "Medicine among the Ancient Hebrews." *Annals of Medical History* 4, no. 3 (May 1942): 219–235.

"Proceedings of the Second International Symposium on Medicine in Bible and Talmud, Jerusalem, December 18–20, 1984." *Koroth* 9, no. 1–2 (special issue). Jerusalem: Israel Institute of Medical History, 1985.

Rosner, Fred. *Medicine in the Mishneh Torah of Maimondes*. New York: KTAV, 1984.

Egypt

Assmann, Jan. *The Mind of Egypt*. New York: Metropolitan Books, 1996.

Brier, Bob. *Ancient Egyptian Magic*. New York: HarperCollins, 1999. First published 1980 by William Morrow (New York).

Bryan, Cyril P. *Ancient Egyptian Medicine: The Papyrus Ebers*. Translated from the German by Cyril P. Bryan. With an introduction by G. Elliott Smith. Chicago: Ares Press, 1974.

Caton, Richard. "I. I-em-hotep and Ancient Egyptian Medicine, II. Prevention of Vascular Disease." The Harveian Oration, June 21, 1904. London: C. J. Clay and Sons, 1904.

Dawson, Warren R. *The Beginnings: Egypt and Assyria.* Clio Medica 1. New York: P. B. Hoeber, 1930.

Fowler, Barbara Hughes, trans. *Love Lyrics of Ancient Egypt.* Chapel Hill: University of North Carolina Press, 1994.

Kemp, Barry. *How to Read the Egyptian Book of the Dead.* New York: W. W. Norton, 2008.

Malaise, Michel. *Les Scarabées de coeur dans l'Égypte ancienne.* Monographies Reine Élisabeth 4. Brussels: Fondation Égyptologique Reine Élisabeth, 1978.

Simpson, William Kelly. *The Literature of Ancient Egypt.* New Haven: Yale University Press, 1972.

Watts, Sheldon. *Disease and Medicine in World History.* New York: Routledge, 2003.

Willerson, James T., and Rebecca Teaff. "Egyptian Contributions to Cardiovascular Medicine." *Texas Heart Institute Journal* 23, no. 3 (1996): 191–200.

Mesopotamia

Avalos, Hector. *Health Care and the Rise of Christianity.* Peabody, MA: Hendrickson, 1999.

Finkel, Irving L., and Markham J. Geller, eds. *Disease in Babylonia.* Cuneiform Monographs 36. Leiden: Brill, 2007.

Geller, Markham J. *Ancient Babylonian Medicine: Theory and Practice.* Chichester: Wiley-Blackwell, 2010.

Leick, Gwendolyn. *The Babylonians: An Introduction.* London: Routledge, 2003.

Meador, Betty De Shong, ed. *Inanna: Lady of Largest Heart: Poems of the Sumerian High Priestess Enheduanna.* Austin: University of Texas Press, 2000.

Oppenheim, A. Leo. "Mesopotamian Medicine." *Bulletin of the History of Medicine* 36, no. 2 (March–April 1962): 97–108.

Parker, Simon B., ed. *Ugaritic Narrative Poetry.* Society of Biblical Literature, Writings from the Ancient World, vol. 9. Atlanta: Scholars Press, 1997.

Sandars, Nancy, ed. *Poems of Heaven and Hell from Ancient Mesopotamia.* New York: Penguin, 1971.

Greek and Roman Medicine

Allbutt, T. Clifford. *Greek Medicine in Rome: The FitzPatrick Lectures on the History of Medicine Delivered at the Royal College of Physicians of London in 1909–1910 with other historical essays.* London: Macmillan, 1921.

Brock, Arthur J., trans. *Greek Medicine: Being Extracts Illustrative of Medical Writers from Hippocrates to Galen.* London: J. M. Dent and Sons, 1929.

Doueihi, Milad. *A Perverse History of the Human Heart.* Cambridge, MA: Harvard University Press, 1997.

Elliott, James Sands. *Outlines of Greek and Roman Medicine.* Boston: Milford House, 1971. First published 1914 by W. Wood (New York).

Harris, C. R. S. *The Heart and the Vascular System in Ancient Greek Medicine from Alcmaeon to Galen*. Oxford: Clarendon Press, 1973.

Horace. *The Complete Works of Horace: The 120 Odes and 42 Longer Poems*. New York: Modern Library, 1936.

Hughes, Jessica. *Votive Body Parts in Greek and Roman Religion*. Cambridge Classical Studies. Cambridge: Cambridge University Press, 2017.

King, Helen. *Greek and Roman Medicine*. Classical World Series. London: Bristol Classical Press, 2001.

Lloyd, G. E. R. *Greek Science after Aristotle*. New York: W. W. Norton, 1973.

Lund, Fred. *Greek Medicine*. Clio Medica 18. New York: P. B. Hoeber, 1936.

Majno, Guido. *The Healing Hands: Man and Wound in the Ancient World*. Cambridge, MA: Harvard University Press, 1975.

Penfield, Wilder. *The Torch*. Boston: Little, Brown, 1960.

Phillips, E. D. *Aspects of Greek Medicine*. New York: St. Martin's Press, 1973.

Sappho. *Sappho: A New Translation*. Translated by Mary Barnard. Oakland: University of California Press, 1958.

Scarborough, John. *Roman Medicine*. Ithaca: Cornell University Press, 1969.

Singer, Charles. *A Short History of Anatomy and Physiology from the Greeks to Harvey*. New York: Dover, 1957.

———. *Greek Biology and Greek Medicine*. Oxford: Clarendon Press, 1922.

The Medieval Heart

Hartnell, Jack. *Medieval Bodies: Life, Death and Art in the Middle Ages.* First published 2018 by Profile Books with Wellcome Collection (London). New York: W. W. Norton, 2019.

Jager, Eric. *The Book of the Heart.* Chicago: University of Chicago Press, 2000.

Webb, Heather. *The Medieval Heart.* New Haven: Yale University Press, 2010.

Islamic Medicine

Abdul Latif, Shifaulmulk Hakim. "Introduction to 'Heart Drugs': A Brilliant Work of Research by Avicenna." In *Avicenna Commemoration Volume*, edited by the Iran Society, 245–254. Kolkata: Iran Society, 1956.

Browne, E. G. *Arabian Medicine: Being the FitzPatrick Lectures Delivered at the College of Physicians in November 1919 and November 1920.* Cambridge: Cambridge University Press, 1962.

Budge, E. A. Wallis, trans. *Syrian Anatomy, Pathology and Therapeutics or "The Book of Medicines."* Volume 1, *Introduction, Syriac Texts.* London: Oxford University Press, 1913.

Campbell, Donald. *Arabian Medicine and Its Influence on the Middle Ages.* Vol. 1. London: Kegan Paul, Trench, Trubner, 1926.

Chatard, J. A. "Avicenna and Arabian Medicine." *Bulletin of the Johns Hopkins Hospital* 19, no. 207 (June 1908): 157–160.

Pormann, Peter E., and Emilie Savage-Smith. *Medieval Islamic Medicine.* Washington, DC: Georgetown University Press, 2007.

Ullmann, Manfred. *Islamic Medicine.* Islamic Surveys 11. Edinburgh: Edinburgh University Press, 1978.

Ancient Indian Medicine

Sharma, J. N. "Cardiovascular System and Its Diseases in Ancient Indian Literature." *Indian Journal of Chest Diseases* 9, no. 1 (January 1967): 32–40.

Sigerist, Henry E. *Early Greek, Hindu, and Persian Medicine.* Vol. 2 of *A History of Medicine.* New York: Oxford University Press, 1961.

Surdas. *Sur's Ocean: Poems from the Early Tradition.* Edited by Kenneth E. Bryant. Translated by John Stratton Hawley. Murty Classical Library of India 5. Cambridge, MA: Harvard University Press, 2015.

Watts, Sheldon. *Disease and Medicine in World History.* New York: Routledge, 2003.

Mesoamerica and the American Indians

Aguilar-Moreno, Manuel. *Handbook to Life in the Aztec World.* First published in 2006 by Facts on File (New York). Oxford: Oxford University Press, 2007.

Bendersky, Gordon. "The Olmec Heart Effigy: Earliest Image of the Human Heart." *Perspectives in Biology and Medicine* 40, no. 3 (Spring 1997): 348–361.

Bray, Warwick. *Everyday Life of the Aztecs.* New York: Dorset Press, 1968.

Domenici, David. *The Aztecs: History and Treasures of an Ancient Civilization.* Vercelli, Italy: White Star Publishers, 2007.

Frazer, James George. *The Golden Bough: A Study in Magic and Religion*. New York: Collier Books, 1922.

Gates, William. *An Aztec Herbal: The Classic Codex of 1552*. Baltimore: Maya Society, 1939. Reprinted with an introduction by Bruce Byland. Mineola, NY: Dover Publications, 2000.

Laughlin, Robert M. *Mayan Hearts*. Illustrated by Naúl Ojeda. Chiapas, Mexico: Taller Leñateros, 2003.

Prescott, William H. *History of the Conquest of Mexico*. 3 vols. New York: Harper and Brothers, 1843.

————. *History of the Conquest of Peru*. 2 vols. New York: Harper and Brothers, 1847.

Schendel, Gordon. *Medicine in Mexico: From Aztec Herbs to Betatrons*. In collaboration with José Alvarez Almézquita and Miguel E. Bustamante. Austin: University of Texas Press, 1968.

Serrato-Combe, Antonio. *The Aztec Templo Mayor: A Visualization*. Salt Lake City: University of Utah Press, 2001.

Stone, Eric. *Medicine Among the American Indians*. Edited by E. B. Krumbhaar. Clio Medica 7. New York: P. B. Hoeber, 1932.

Supernant, Kisha, Jane Eva Baxter, Natasha Lyons, and Sonya Atalay, eds. *Archaeologies of the Heart*. Cham, Switzerland: Springer Nature Switzerland, 2020. See especially chapter 16 "An Archaeology Led by Strawberries" by Sonya Atalay, 253–269.

Eastern Asian Medicine

Harris, Peter, ed. *Zen Poems*. Everyman's Library edition. New York: Alfred A. Knopf, 1999.

Horine, Emmet Field. "An Epitome of Ancient Pulse Lore." *Bulletin of the History of Medicine* 10, no. 2 (July 1941): 209–249.

Lock, Margaret M. *East Asian Medicine in Urban Japan*. Berkeley: University of California Press, 1980.

MacMillan, Peter, trans. *One Hundred Poets, One Poem Each: A Treasure of Classical Japanese Verse*. New York: Penguin, 2018.

Needham, Joseph. *Science and Civilization in China*. Cambridge, UK: Cambridge University Press, 1954.

Shi Jizong, and Chu Feng Zhu. *The ABC of Traditional Chinese Medicine*. Translated by Shi Jiaxin. Hong Kong: Hai Feng, 1985.

Unschuld, Paul U. *Medicine in China: A History of Ideas*. Berkeley: University of California Press, 1985.

Van Alphen, Jan, and Anthony Aris, eds. *Oriental Medicine: An Illustrated Guide to the Asian Arts of Healing*. Boston: Shambala, 1996.

Watts, Sheldon. *Disease and Medicine in World History*. New York: Routledge, 2003.

Yu Fujikawa. *Japanese Medicine*. Clio Medica 12. Translated from the German by John Ruräh. New York: P. B. Hoeber, 1934.

Finale

Renfrew, Colin, and Iain Morley, eds. *Image and Imagination: A Global Prehistory of Figurative Representation*. Cambridge, UK: McDonald Institute for Archaeological Research, 2007.

Yonck, Richard. *The Heart of the Machine: Our Future in a World of Artificial Emotional Intelligence*. New York: Arcade, 2017.

General Bibliography

Anati, Emmanuel. *Les Origines de L'Art et La Formation de L'Esprit Humain.* Paris: Albin Michel, 1989.

———. *Origini dell'Arte e della Concettualitá.* Milan: Jaca Book, 1988.

Baines, John, and Jaromir Málek. *Cultural Atlas of Ancient Egypt.* New York: Checkmark Books, 2000.

Berenguer, Magín. *Prehistoric Man and His Art: The Caves of Ribadesella.* Park Ridge, NJ: Noyes Press, 1975.

Boisaubin, Eugene V. "Cardiology in Ancient Egypt." *Texas Heart Institute Journal* 15, no. 2 (1988): 80–85.

Bollettino del Centro Camuno di Studi Preistorici (BCSP). Vol. 27 (1993).

Camac, C. N. B. *Imhotep to Harvey: Backgrounds of Medical History.* New York: P. B. Hoeber, 1931.

Cameron, M. L. *Anglo-Saxon Medicine.* Cambridge Studies in Anglo-Saxon England 7. Cambridge, UK: Cambridge University Press, 1993.

Celsus. *De Medicina.* Translated by W. G. Spencer. Cambridge, MA: Harvard University Press, 1935.

Cunliffe, Barry, ed. *The Oxford Illustrated Prehistory of Europe.* Oxford, UK: Oxford University Press, 1994.

De Puma, Richard Daniel, and Jocelyn Penny Small, eds. *Murlo and the Etruscans: Art and Society in Ancient Eruria.* Madison: University of Wisconsin Press, 1994. See especially the chapter "Anatomical Votives and Italian Medical Traditions" by Jean MacIntosh Turfa, 224–240.

East, Terence. *The Story of Heart Disease: The FitzPatrick Lectures for 1956 and 1957 Given before the Royal College of Physicians in London.* London: William Dawson and Sons, 1958.

End, Adelheid, and Ernst Wolner. "The Heart: Location of the Human Soul, Site of Surgical Intervention." *Journal of Cardiac Surgery* 8, no. 3 (May 1993): 398–403.

Estes, J. Worth. *The Medical Skills of Ancient Egypt.* Canton, MA: Science History Publications/USA, 1989.

Fernández, Justino. *Mexican Art.* Photographs by Constantino Reges-Valerio. The Colour Library of Art. London: Paul Hamlyn, 1967.

Furley, David J., and J. S. Wilkie. *Galen: On Respiration and the Arteries.* Princeton: Princeton University Press, 1984.

Garrison, Fielding H. *An Introduction to the History of Medicine.* 8 vols. Philadelphia: Saunders, 1914.

Haddad, Sami I., and Amin A. Khairallah. "A Forgotten Chapter in the History of the Circulation of the Blood." *Annals of Surgery* 104, no. 1 (July 1936): 1–8.

Hamburger, Walter W. "The Earliest Known Reference to the Heart and Circulation: The Edwin Smith Surgical Papyrus, circa 3000 BC." *American Heart Journal* 17, no. 3 (March 1939): 259–274.

Herrick, James B. *A Short History of Cardiology.* Springfield, IL: Charles C. Thomas, 1942.

Hillier, S. M., and J. A. Jewell. *Heath Care and Traditional Medicine in China, 1800–1982.* London: Routledge and Keegan Paul, 1983.

Innes, Hammond. *The Conquistadors.* New York: Alfred A. Knopf, 1969.

Jackson, Ralph. *Doctors and Diseases in the Roman Empire*. Norman: University of Oklahoma Press, 1988.

Jayne, Walter Addison. *The Healing Gods of Ancient Civilizations*. New Haven: Yale University Press, 1925.

Potter, T. W., and Calvin Wells. "A Republican Healing-Sanctuary at Ponte di Nona near Rome and the Classical Tradition of Votive Medicine." *Journal of the British Archaeological Association* 138 (1985): 23–47.

Ruspoli, Mario. *The Cave of Lascaux: The Final Photographs*. New York: Harry Abrams, 1987.

Sarton, George. *Galen of Pergamon*. Logan Clendening Lectures on the History and Philosophy of Medicine, 3rd series. Lawrence: University of Kansas Press, 1954.

Sigerist, Henry E. *Primitive and Archaic Medicine*. Vol. 1 of *A History of Medicine*. New York: Oxford University Press, 1951.

Siraisi, Nancy G. "Early Anatomy in Comparative Perspective: Introduction." *Journal of the History of Medicine and Allied Sciences* 50, no. 1 (January 1995): 3–10.

———. *Medieval and Early Renaissance Medicine: An Introduction to Knowledge and Practice*. Chicago: University of Chicago Press, 1990.

Sten, María. *Codices of Mexico and Their Extraordinary History*. Mexico: Panorama Editorial, 1979.

Taylor, Henry Osborn. *Greek Biology and Medicine*. Our Debt to Greece and Rome. Series edited by George D. Hadzits and David M. Robinson. New York: Cooper Square Publishers, 1963.

Ucko, Peter J., and Andrée Rosenfeld. *Paleolithic Cave Art*. World University Library series. New York: McGraw-Hill, 1967.

Von Hagan, Victor Wolfgang. *The Ancient Sun Kingdoms of the Americas.* London: Paladin, 1977.

Zimmerman, M. R. "The Paleopathology of the Cardiovascular Systems." *Texas Heart Institute Journal* 20, no. 4 (1993): 252–257.

ACKNOWLEDGMENTS

I am a physician—not an historian, theologian, or literary writer. So, I am indebted to those who helped me make this essay a reality:

John Greenebaum, Noah Grey, and Allan Weiss for advice and corrections,

Emma Aprile, my editor, who made this essay a little more readable,

and Fisher Nash, who negotiated publishing hurdles with me.

Finally, and most importantly, the guidance of my wife, Terry, also a physician, made possible this final product.

ABOUT THE AUTHOR

Dr. Morris Weiss Jr. graduated from the University of Louisville School of Medicine in 1958, has specialty boards in internal medicine and cardiology, and just completed on June 28, 2022, his sixtieth year in practice.

Printed in the United States
by Baker & Taylor Publisher Services